BRAIN EVANGELISTS

How Psychiatry Has Convinced Us to Believe in Its Far-Fetched Science and Dubious Treatments

BRAIN EVANGELISTS

GORDON WARME, MD

UAC PRESS

UAC Press
Toronto, Canada

Cataloguing in Publication Data available
from Library and Archives Canada

ISBN 978-0-9951906-0-3 (paperback)
ISBN 978-0-9951906-1-0 (ebook)

Cover and text design by Peter Cocking
Editing by Arlene Prunkl
Proofreading by Lana Okerland
Printed and bound in the United States

16 17 18 19 20 5 4 3 2 1

Contents

ALSO BY GORDON WARME

Reluctant Treasures: The Practice of Analytic Psychotherapy

The Psychotherapist: The Use and Abuse of Psychological Influence

The Cure of Folly: A Psychiatrist's Cautionary Tale

Daggers of the Mind: The Myth of Mental Illness

. . . a feeling of profound melancholy came over him in his survey of the bustling place. There is a great quantity of eating and drinking, making love and jilting, laughing and the contrary, smoking, cheating, fighting, dancing, and fiddling: there are bullies pushing about, bucks ogling the women, knaves picking pockets . . . quacks (*other* quacks, plague take them!) bawling in front of their booths . . .. Yes, this is VANITY FAIR; not a moral place certainly; nor a merry one, though very noisy.

W.M. THACKERAY, *Vanity Fair* (Prologue)

Introduction

My self-confidence as a guru had gone.
ARTHUR KOESTLER,
lapsed Communist, author, journalist

I'VE ALWAYS AIMED to be normal. I've worked hard, earned money, made friends, and remembered birthdays. But in May of 2015 I forgot the birthdays of Mariah and Alex, two of my grandchildren, and even more embarrassingly, the birthdays of two of my children, Diana and Paul. If four important birthdays occur in one month they're hard to forget, and the truth is they hadn't completely slipped my mind. Since I have no signs of Alzheimer's, I can't be let off the hook, nor do I have any of the disorders invented by my psychiatric colleagues that supposedly cause forgetfulness and that could bring forgiveness—attention deficit, perhaps, or some wearisome stress problem. I'd *neglected* the birthdays, failed to attend and focus. I know what was going on: I was writing this book. I was cunningly negligent, living out a romantic stereotype that included not shaving, dropping clothes to the floor, and not phoning friends.

I'm an artist wannabe.

A real artist can turn anything into art. She doesn't simply talk with friends or fix her hair, nor does she only paint portraits or direct plays. She watches. "I am a camera," said Christopher Isherwood. When in the throes of love—romantic, ecstatic love—most of us pick up the thousand artistic nuances of what's going on, and nuance is what the psychiatrist is after. Not success, not accomplishment, but savouring a detail, a turn of phrase, brilliant touches, eye-play, a smile or a tear. Because she's become half-hearted about these things, the modern psychiatrist hasn't been doing a good job of tapping into her artistic and poetic talents and has ended up depriving her patients of the best thing she does. Sensational reports about psychiatric discoveries, science, and soon-to-arrive cures guarantee that some people will be surprised by my emphasis on the artistic and the poetic. It's more than a surprise for me. Once I'd digested the idea that to do her work properly the psychiatrist must call on her own artistry, I became more and more frustrated by how my profession operates.

Yes, I'm worrying about psychiatry. On this trip to Mexico, I'm determined to finish this book, all the while on the lookout for cultural enthrallments, traditions different from mine that I hope will stir me up, stimulate me. Among other things, I'll check out the shamans in San Juan Chamula I saw twenty years ago, whom I then didn't take seriously enough. What I'm upset about is that my colleagues, without evidence, demean our patients, unthinkingly saying they have abnormal chemicals in their brains or that their personalities are abnormal, twisted, then given horrible names like *borderline*, *narcissistic*, and *infantile*. The truth is that we psychiatrists have access to no objective findings; our patients' social practices our only source of information. We therefore must attend carefully to their speeches, actions, and favourite metaphors, collect biographical information, and ponder their odd opinions and vain or self-insulting talk—very different from the type of information collected by other doctors.

Surgeons, family doctors, and other non-psychiatric medical specialists zero in on material abnormalities in their patients' organs, bodies, and brains. Then, through rational effort and experiment, real diseases are discovered, studied, and often cured—very different from what's done by doctors like me. Since no tangible abnormalities exist in psychiatric patients ("abnormal brain chemicals" and "psychological complexes" are the delusions of those who tell us about them, delusions caused, I assume, by "abnormal chemicals" in their brains), we psychiatrists tackle the problem of cure and change differently from other doctors—we have no choice but to put language and images at centre stage. If I change metaphors, do the problems of psychiatric patients look different? How will you react if, instead of "disease," I say of my patient that he has a tragic, worrisome, or bizarre way of life? If I get poetic and say that he lives according to the rules of a different god, will you think I'm a fool, or will that new metaphor cast a different light on things? If, instead of saying he has an affliction, I announce that my patient presents himself to the world in a strange, shocking, or unhappy way, might that get you thinking, or because this is a touchy subject, will you send me to hell?

I have to be careful, especially because I'm going to own up to something else that will be controversial: most psychiatric cures are due to the placebo effect, an effect that is a subcategory of human bewitchments like falling in love, not stepping on the cracks in the sidewalk, idealizing monstrous leaders like Mao Tse-tung, and shrieking or fainting at a rock concert. It doesn't matter whether we call it a cultural practice, mass hysteria, or the placebo effect: what it boils down to is superstition.

Non-psychiatric doctors, on the other hand, can count on hard-nosed science to discover and to cure real diseases, a fact so obvious that there's no need for them to trumpet their scientific credentials. Insiders like me aren't supposed to let you in on such secrets, but when a psychiatrist talks about science it's out of insecurity, out of habit, or as public relations. If you ask them about science, many of my colleagues won't think carefully about your question; they will carelessly say that, yes, of course there is scientific knowledge about the causes of psychiatric problems, and they'll make vague references to genes, brain functions, and abnormal chemicals. If *I*, a member of the profession, tease such a psychiatrist about this when I run into her outside my office ("Come on, Sandra, give me the skinny about the biological causes of schizophrenia"), she'll answer differently, nearly always with an awkward chuckle, and will dither: "Well, we're getting close…"; "There is 'suggestive evidence' (they love that phrase) that…" I'm most bothered when my colleagues answer quasi-religiously, give me a faith-based answer: "There *must* be a biological abnormality that causes schizophrenia" (analogously: "There *must* be an intelligent design that caused the world to come into existence"). Psychiatrists are touchy about these things, so I have to be careful; alienating colleagues is a waste of time. Yet it will take more than a nudge and a wink to get my colleagues to notice: as I write this book, I'll call on all the strength and determination I've got to make my case.

I'M A TALKING doctor. There are dozens of psychotherapies, but like most talking doctors, I stick to my own preferred ways. Nowadays, many of my colleagues give medications, and for them the cornucopia of drugs they can choose from comes in *tens* of dozens. Others give shock treatments and, alarmingly, some even stick needles into their patients' heads to do something called deep-brain stimulation. We're a bit like a drugstore with hundreds of over-the-counter cough medicines on sale that don't do much (when treating patients with chest diseases, hospital doctors rarely prescribe cough medicine). As has been true since history began, the so-called treatments administered by alienists—psychiatrists, shamans, herbalists, and other cultists—are cultural artifacts, the current fashion, symbolic stabs in the dark that are comforting to patients, but that change no disease process: they are placebos. As a student in various countries, I went along with the then-current placebos: mustard plasters for pneumonia (England), *Herring Salat* as a bowel preparation before a sigmoidoscopy (Germany), an antidepressant regime based on menial work (USA), and insulin coma for schizophrenia (Canada). Until 150 years ago, nearly all of medicine was hokey, most medical practices being nothing more than similar stabs in the dark, sometimes cruel, as in this passage from *Nikolai Gogol*, Nabokov's short biography of Gogol.

> Dr. Auvers . . . had his patient plunged into a warm bath where his head was soused with cold water after which he was put to bed with half-a-dozen plump leeches affixed to his nose. He had groaned and weakly struggled while his wretched body (you could feel the spine through his stomach) was carried to a deep wooden bath; he shivered as he lay naked in bed and kept pleading to have the leeches removed: they were dangling from his nose and getting into his mouth . . .

Psychiatrists haven't noticed that the rest of medicine has given up on such foolishness—on herring salads and humours and leeches and bleeding and purging—and also haven't noticed that, because they have unmistakable biological abnormalities, non-psychiatric patients are fundamentally different from psychiatric patients. This is not to say that modern psychiatrists are neglectful. On the contrary, psychiatrists work hard—and each works differently. But if psychiatrists can't get straight what they're doing, why keep this up? Despite good feedback, it's clear that psychiatrists are spinning their wheels. Freud, busy discovering complexes, rapes, and fantasies, was also possessed by a gruesome earnestness.

Like our predecessors—priests, shamans, gurus, and medicine men or women—we are caught, stuck with theories of abnormal brains that have been around for millennia, frantic to squeeze the odd messages sent out by our unhappy and unconventional patients into simple formulas such as "schizophrenia is caused by a schizophrenia gene, a schizophrenia chemical, a schizophrenia lesion, or a schizophrenia principle." That's a bit like saying hatred is caused by a hatred principle and sleep by a dormitive principle. Silly though such theories are, politics trumps facts every time, most recently the politics of research funding to investigate diseases that don't exist. As far back as history goes, when a person's oddness has been extreme enough (nowadays psychiatrists label them schizophrenic), we in Western society have persuaded ourselves that our patients are exceptional in one of five ways:

- Believed to have abnormal brains as far back as history goes.
- Said to have imbalances of certain substances in the body: the four elements (air, fire, water, and earth) in ancient times, later re-named as four humours (black bile, yellow bile, phlegm, and blood), re-named yet again as abnormal chemicals (no current suspects) in the twentieth and twenty-first centuries.
- They are gods: Jesus, the Pythia at Delphi, Father Divine, Reverend Jim Jones of Jonestown infamy.
- They are possessed by demons, witches, or devils that must be released from the head by trepanation, burped out when a Mexican

shaman gives them Coca-Cola to drink, and, even in 2016, to be evicted by a Catholic or Anglican priest through exorcism.

- They have traumatic memories that must be exposed or eliminated, emotions that must be "expressed," and sins that must be confessed.

If we look closely, the only thing to be seen in a psychiatric patient is unhappy or strange talk and actions. When we "solve" the problem of odd behaviour by using the language of disease and treatment, we end up doing experiments that are useless, sometimes benign, at other times harmful, experiments abandoned after a few years only to be replaced by new potions and procedures, practices just as wrongheaded as those tried before. We're caught in a set of superstitions that are full cousins to superstitions that we rightfully scorn: treating a child's leukemia with a preposterous diet; surgically removing imaginary vascular obstructions from the necks of people with multiple sclerosis; attributing bizarre thinking to satanic possession. Maybe I should listen to more optimistic news items, get cracking on enthusiasms that, according to some media reports, definitely work: a diet reported on in this morning's *Globe and Mail*; L. Ron Hubbard's *Dianetics*; proper sleep hygiene; being reborn in Christ; and, I now realize, certain versions of psychiatry, a cutting-edge psychotherapeutic method, or an upgraded psychoactive drug—nobody knows which one.

Although some think the psychiatric enterprise will collapse any day, for now, psychiatry goes from one self-deluded triumph to another. Sadly, by ignoring the rules of science, it's a cinch for researchers to fool themselves and the public because, all too often, hope wins out over nasty facts.[1] Yes, researchers believe so strongly in what they are doing that they fool even themselves. In chapter 8 I'll discuss the rules of science that, were they followed, would expose psychiatric research to be a house of cards, showing that psychiatric "discoveries" don't exist and can't exist.

---

1 Jerry Adler, "The Reformation: Can Social Scientists Save Themselves?" *Pacific Standard: The Science of Society* (April 28, 2014). http://www.psmag.com/health-and-behavior/can-social-scientists-save-themselves-human-behavior-78858.

EVERY ERA AND every culture has a system in place that, when a person is upset, allows him to talk to an expert. That expert, be she[2] a psychiatrist, priest, or shaman, responds by talking, giving a potion, invoking a ritual, or often all three—for example, psychotherapy, swallowing an antidepressant pill, and lying on a couch; confessing to a priest, swallowing the body and blood of Christ, and prostrating oneself before the cross. What these things accomplish is quite another matter. These days, when I think I have an answer, I'm suspicious—*very* suspicious—because the complex of words, signs, and messages given off by patients is so complicated that I'm at risk of glomming onto a spurious medical treatment or a silly "awakening" or "rebirth" fantasy, things as futile as New Year's resolutions. Miserable patients want to talk, and some need more than that—a nudge or a firm push, because, even though they want to change, patients are also strangely obstinate; many fight to *not* change. Psychiatrists are important in every culture, even when they carry a different label: priest, guru, shaman, imam, rabbi, witch doctor, medicine man or woman.

Many years ago I was a resident at the Hospital for Sick Children in Toronto, where I worked for Bill Mustard, the tough-minded chief surgeon of the cardiac surgery unit. Mustard was notorious for giving his residents a hard time, but once he and I got to know each other, he seemed to be easier on me than on others who'd worked for him. Because he knew I intended to become a psychiatrist, when he did torment me, he took a special delight in it. "Don't waste your time psychologizing," he would say. "Buckle down, make diagnoses, and use your head; anything else is for lazy poets and sissies." Once I became a psychiatrist, I disobeyed—I buckled down and tried to use my head to think *with the vigour and determination of a tough-minded surgeon*, attending to poetics and semantics I'd not before noticed.

"At seventy-seven, it's time to be in earnest," said Samuel Johnson. Since I'm older than that, I'm overdue. Although long-winded, my argument isn't mysterious: to explain psychiatry is to take on human life—love, tragedy, humour, and all the rest. Were this a novel, a

---

2 When possible, I refer to the doctor as *she* and to the patient as *he*. The names of patients have been changed.

short story, or a poem, it might achieve the same thing as my logic and evidence.

A warning: every person I describe herein is contradictory, a mishmash, a collage, so don't be surprised if I sometimes leave you up in the air, try to persuade you that incoherence and inconclusiveness are part of every person, part of every story that is told, and part of many of my chapters. As a book about psychiatry should do, I want this book to persuade you to think.

And before I even begin, I offer two conclusions:

Everything is biography.

Everyone has experiences with teachers, priests, imams, and medicine men and women.

PART ONE

HELPING PEOPLE

1

A Helping Hand, a Pill or Two, and Thoughtfulness

If you're going through hell, keep going.
WINSTON CHURCHILL

IN 1943, MY Aunt Dona was having trouble. She complained that other passengers on streetcars were staring at her, and at her work place, everyone criticized her. She decided that a streetcar conductor was gossiping about her, and she made a scene bad enough that he had to stop his trolley and shoo her out onto the street. She spent a lot of time at our house, most of the time arguing and accusing. One day, Dr. Broad, our family doctor, was making a house call because someone was sick, so my mother told him about Dona's troubles. "Well," he said. "She needs a break. Doesn't she have a sister in Halifax she's close to? Tell her I said she's to take a couple of weeks off work and go to stay with her sister." We all knew that Dona and her sister Rosie often argued, but Dona nevertheless went. After two weeks of bickering with her sister, she came back to Toronto, her suspicious paranoia gone.

Dr. Broad was wily and experienced.

MANY WHO COME to hospitals are not fully mad. They get better, some quickly, cured by pills, talk, or other medical magic—by drugs that really work, and by an array of symbolic interventions. Sometimes their stories are benign, with happy endings, but others are unchangeable tragedies. If questioned closely, all patients have stories that are dramatic and complicated, even if the urgent clinic is too busy for anyone to flush out the details; mostly, there's no time to storm the citadel or to re-dream someone's life. About her way of working with these patients, my ideal psychiatrist admits the truth: she has ready at hand a set of gestures she's become skilled at using and can tailor to suit a particular patient. She wishes she had time to discover and discuss the unique life story of every person who comes to the clinic, but she hasn't. On the front line, the psychiatrist relies mostly on relationship cures and placebo cures, the cures promised by psychiatrists and that give people hope. Briefly and temporarily, to get them through a rough patch, she also gives drugs.

All psychiatrists ought to spend time working with urgent cases. Not only that, we talking doctors ought to see more deeply disturbed patients in our own offices, brushing up on how to use the drugs that, even though overused, are sometimes necessary to give short-term relief. Just like everyone else, we deceive ourselves with excuses for why we sit in our offices seeing only more culturally adroit patients, those well enough to search out fancy doctors (me, for example), those interested in soul-searching and serious talk. We humans are stubbornly ourselves, determined to pursue our well-established ways. Changing human behaviour, social systems, and cultural institutions is a forbidding project, so a stubborn, counter-determination is necessary, a resolve or will to do things differently—while remaining calm. I was at a bullfight here in Mexico City yesterday and came away with the idea that I am calm like a matador who, grim-faced, makes passionate love with his bull, to whom he ardently calls out, "*Toro! Toro bravo!*"

Most patients, those with mental aches, common wounds, fears, and silliness, reward the psychiatrist with praise and testimonials no matter what she does—all it takes is a pill or two, a bit of talk with a confident doctor. If the patient feels better, his gratitude is justified, but since everyday life is more scripted than we think, that gratitude is also archetypal—like most of us, the patient has been brought up to be grateful and admiring of his doctor, and that gratitude, often intense, ought to be one of the things the psychiatrist is suspicious of. Instead, her patient's praise leads the psychiatrist into temptation, lures her into thinking she may be a wizard, that she is special; she risks forgetting that she is a cultural institution, that awe and admiration of the doctor/guru figure is part of every culture. She must remind herself that she has other patients, the envious, greedy, and paranoid, pessimists and whiners who scorn her and her ilk and are resistant, baffling, and ungrateful. Because she doesn't cure them, these patients wreck everything. She is therefore tempted to reassign them to a category that fits with certain bad psychiatric habits, to label them *unsuitable*, *resistant*, or *noncompliant*.

What follows are three case histories, stories from the lives of three people: one from the emergency department (Georges Valois), one from the outpatient clinic (Jake Andrews), and one from my private practice (Janice Brittain). My intent is to familiarize you with the shape of a psychiatrist's day, what she struggles with, and how she deals with the problems that come her way. You will notice that only with the second case is there serious psychiatric talk. With the first and third cases, the task was simply to get someone through a rough patch.

Georges Valois: The police brought Mr. Valois, cursing and struggling, to the emergency department in restraints. The staff tried to reassure him that he would be all right, but when they released him, he struck out at whoever was closest. His face was purple with rage, his veins stood out as he struggled, and he spat at anyone who talked to him. He had been brought from a fitness club, where he had attacked a spinning instructor. The staff of the club told the police that Mr. Valois was a regular at spinning classes, but the instructor had recently noticed him muttering under his breath during the classes. That day, partway through the class, the instructor had spoken to him. "Are you okay, Georges?"

Mr. Valois didn't answer. He put his head down and pedalled harder, not looking up for the remainder of the class. When the class was over, he waited until everyone had left and then spoke angrily to the instructor: "Why did you ask me how I was? Why did you single me out? What kind of a patronizing asshole are you?" The instructor explained that he liked him and was worried about him.

"You fucking prick. See, you're doing it again, thinking there's something wrong with me." And when the instructor tried to reassure him further, Mr. Valois shoved him hard, and they fought. Several club members helped hold Mr. Valois down, the police were called, and because he seemed incoherent and confused, he was brought to the hospital. The staff noticed that when they tried to reassure him, he responded just as he had at the fitness club: he became even more furious. Against his will, Mr. Valois was injected with the drug haloperidol. After half an hour, no calmer, he was given another injection of the same drug. Although calmer, later that evening Mr. Valois still seemed confused, but agreed to be admitted to the hospital's short-term care unit.

The next day, he explained that although he had never before been physically aggressive, he had a temper. Because he was sure that he was by then okay, and with the agreement of the doctor, he went home with a three-day prescription for lorazepam and an appointment to see the doctor a week later. At that appointment, he expressed regret for the trouble he had caused, explaining that he had written an apology to the spinning instructor, and that, as someone on the psychiatric unit had suggested, he would think about attending anger management classes. The doctor wasn't sure whether Mr. Valois was telling the truth.

I'm unpopular if I insist that removing someone's civil rights is a moral decision, not a medical one—but it is, and only the law should legislate morality. A psychiatrist is in flawed moral territory if she thinks a person should be detained because he upsets his family, friends, doctors, or the police. If my wife upsets me, should she be locked up against her will? What if she screams at me? Throws dishes? And me . . . should I be locked up if I punch a hole in the wall, shout at my wife, and call her a bitch in front of my children? In the clinic, the psychiatrist should confine herself to calming the patient, not according to a protocol, a manual, or formal criteria, but using common sense—the common sense that's always liable to misfire, yet it is the only thing we've got to go by. Any actions beyond immediate and urgent comforting—with drugs or with words—should not be allowed, certainly nothing that would allow the psychiatrist to confine someone like Mr. Valois against his will. Despite my smug confidence that there'd be no problem were it me (the all-knowing and always sensible "me") making these decisions, it's wrong that, because I'm a psychiatrist, the law has given me that power.

We psychiatrists need to monitor ourselves, think harder about our actions. It's our duty to permit individuals to invent themselves as they wish; since coercion is primarily a legal and police matter, even if a law is broken our task is to avoid coercive measures whenever possible. With Mr. Valois, violent and incoherent, it's best to act informally and take him to a hospital—as the police did. There, because things often clear up, he can eat, snooze, talk things over, stay for a few nights. Despite our nervousness about how he will fare, he can then go his own way. Never mind that we psychiatrists worry about being sued if things don't go well; surely it's safe to do sensible things, to let Mr. Valois go his way even if a risk exists that something might go wrong. These are commonplace risks, far smaller than driving on a highway.

Obviously things don't always clear up. Mr. Valois could have turned out to be quite crazy even if no longer confused. (I've run into policies that forbid the use of the word *crazy*, even though that word is far better than weasel words like *schizophrenia* and *bipolar*. *Mad* is also better, just as *dead* is better than *passed on* and *eternal rest*, *affair* and *adultery* better than *fooling around*.) And if he is crazy, it's harder to decide what to do. But if he insists on going his own way, most of the time we ought to just let him go.

Jake Andrews: Until he came to the clinic in 2009, Mr. Andrews hadn't noticed that the bad marriage he complained of resembled his parents' marriage, that his father had failed to be a good husband in the same way Mr. Andrews was failing to be a good husband. During the interview, he realized that in an odd way *his* failed marriage took the edge off his father's marital failure; how could he think ill of his father if he had done no better? And when during his second appointment Mr. Andrews said, "Marriage is a pile of crap," he suddenly had a thought that caught his attention: "I'm doing it again. I'm saying that my father doesn't deserve any fault at all; the fault is in the institution of marriage itself."

The interpretation of his behaviour in our conversation wasn't a discovery of facts not previously known. It was just a way of putting his life together that made sense in the particular conversation we were having. Although Mr. Andrews's new observations were signs of change, they were not signs that a disease had been cured. He'd learned something. And once a patient has learned something, he is different. Trivial? Perhaps. But if patients think such things over, differences become contagious, infect other habits of thought. It's like discovering a hotel charge on your husband's credit card—there's a contagion effect, and things that once seemed innocent add up differently. Those evening meetings he goes to now become suspect.

Parallels are both embraced and denied: "I'm my father, but I'm definitely not my father." Mr. Andrews didn't realize how similar his marriage was to his parents' marriage, but at the same time, he understood the almost perfect parallel. This ambiguity in human behaviour, knowing and not knowing at the same time, makes it impossible to apply a scientific method to human behaviour, be it mad, normal, benign, or screwball. Nor will the ambiguity ever explain my behaviour—my behaviour that to me is so obviously "normal." Science depends on reliable findings, replicable data, and in psychiatry such things don't exist. Some will say that there's lots of ambiguity in quantum physics. But in quantum physics, the findings are replicable, and although I don't understand the mathematics, the findings are also predictable.

Had it been recommended, I suspect that Mr. Andrews would have come regularly for further appointments, but whether right or wrong, that's not what I suggested. Since he quickly saw patterns in his life he'd not noticed before, I proposed that he think things over, and if in a week or so he decided he wanted to talk further, he could give me a call. I sensed a flicker of disappointment, yet he did not call back.

Later, I worried that I'd been cavalier, that I hadn't given enough credit to him for his decision to come to the clinic, that he'd needed more than two brief meetings. Would he have taken the time to think things over and then changed after those few interviews, as I hoped? Should I have encouraged him to return? No one knows, but I do know that a probing interview—if that was how Mr. Andrews experienced it—gets people thinking. Most of us have had such affecting experiences, often with a teacher. I also know that my recommendation was neither scientifically based nor did it follow a rational protocol. It was my whim, my social intuition of what ought to be done, informed by my training and experience. On other occasions, the recommendation is that a patient should return more often, sometimes for months. But mostly, it ought to be for just a few weeks. Only intuition and judgment are in play, a hunch that a patient's life will either improve or go badly, and in the latter case it's my duty to intervene more strongly in his life than I thought necessary for Mr. Andrews.

A year later, Mr. Andrews *did* phone. He wasn't as worried about his marriage as he had been, but he had a vague sense that he once again needed to talk to someone about his life. We arranged to meet for twenty appointments. Again, he talked about his father, who he now explained was his stepfather. He'd never met his biological father. When he was twelve years old, his mother told him she'd been pregnant with another man's child when she married; until then, he'd thought his stepfather was his real father. Even though his stepfather had been good to him, he suspected that his parents' marital problems had arisen because his stepfather thought of him as an outsider, an intruder, even a threat.

Mr. Andrews was the manager of a supermarket and, as we neared the end of our twenty therapy sessions, a nasty incident occurred at work. There'd been a Christmas party at the head office the night before our appointment. There'd been drinking and hilarity, and a senior person in the company had become the centre of attention, telling ribald stories and encouraging others to join in.

"It was bad," said Mr. Andrews. "Last night at the party, he got all the guys to tell vulgar stories about picking up women in airports and bars, talking about women as though they were sluts, the usual macho bullshit. I was upset they were making fools of themselves, and I could see that this one guy was provoking the whole thing. I'd also had a couple of drinks. Then, suddenly, this senior management guy turned on his colleagues and denounced them for their vulgarity, their unfaithfulness to their wives, and so on. I decided I wouldn't put up with his disgusting behaviour and ended up telling him off right in front of the whole crowd, told him he was a self-righteous prick who'd started the whole thing. I might even have put my job in jeopardy. I don't remember much after that—I was sort of amnesic driving home. It wasn't the booze because I hadn't drunk that much. Even this morning, I was kind of mixed up and couldn't really remember what had happened last night. I couldn't even get clear in my head that I was meeting with you at nine this morning, even though it's our regular time. I finally remembered in the waiting room what had happened."

"Mr. Andrews," I said, "when you told off the troublemaker, who was speaking you?"

"I dunno," he answered, brushing aside my slightly odd question, "but hearing you speak right now, I understand what's going on. It's you I was telling off last night. You're the guy who keeps getting me to tell all my dirty secrets, just like that guy last night that was getting everybody else to tell their dirty secrets. I come here every week and you sit there and let me pour my guts out."

A long silence ensued. Then he went on. "Telling you about the senior guy last night, I was actually furious at *you*, but now it's just disappeared. And I'm having trouble remembering again. I almost forget what I was talking about. But I guess it's clear that I'm mad at you and I took it out on that guy last night. He's senior management and you're sort of senior management."

"Well, Mr. Andrews," I said. "I think the analogy you've discovered is important, but there's another analogy, one that has to do with two fathers. I suspect your biological father and your stepfather are two ghosts, and they lie behind two other ghosts—me and the guy at the party, the two other 'senior management' people."

Four years passed. Then, in 2013, Mr. Andrews called again. "I've been thinking about something. Could I come in and bounce it off you?" When he arrived, he bothered with no preliminaries, not even to say how his life was going. "Do you recall that incident when I told off the senior management guy at the Christmas party? When I told you the story, the first thing you said was something a bit off the wall, 'Who was speaking you?' I don't think I really answered that. And I sort of forgot about it. Then, six weeks ago, I was on a tour bus in Banff and some woman made a racist remark about all the Japanese tourists in the town. The same thing happened as at the Christmas party. I told her off, right in front of the whole busload of people, really nasty and insulting, and wouldn't let her argue back. I figured I'd done the right thing, and maybe I had, but the point is that I was out of control. And I went too far. I wrecked the tour for myself because all the other people in our group were uneasy with me after that. It's not that they liked this woman; everybody'd already taken a dislike to her because she was always complaining, but my nastiness made people feel sorry for her.

"Anyhow, after that, I remembered what you'd said about who was speaking me. In fact, your words kept running through my head repeatedly: 'Who was speaking you?' And all of a sudden, it was obvious. It was my mother. When I get nasty like that, it's her words coming out of my mouth. When I was a kid, she used to do stuff like that in stores, telling people off, and I used to be embarrassed and try to pretend I wasn't with her."

It seemed that with Jake Andrews I'd concentrated on many associations, parallels, links, and analogies, but I hadn't persisted in my important intuitive question, the question about whom he had become, who was speaking with his voice when he blew his stack. Identification, too, is the creation of an analogy: "I'm my mother."

Janice Brittain: Dr. Brittain was also cured, so to speak, mostly by life events and one meeting with me. Her husband, a physiotherapist, had originally suggested that she call me. She practised sports medicine, as did her father. She was a confident woman, and when she strode into my office, her ponytail bounced from side to side.

Married for six months, she and her husband had been quarrelling about their sex life. Her husband, she said, had little interest in sexual intercourse but enjoyed cuddling and joining her in the shower. He also liked her to give him oral sex or to masturbate him. To reciprocate—reluctantly, she thought—he performed a parody of oral sex: rather than doing so with his mouth, he stimulated her with his nose. She had assumed they would eventually work things out, but an incident two weeks before our meeting had unsettled her. In the sports medicine clinic, she'd seen a man with a shoulder injury who she recognized as a fellow she'd dated a few times in high school. At the end of the appointment, they'd chatted briefly and he suggested they meet for coffee to catch up. Since she had only one more appointment that day, they decided to meet downstairs at Tim Horton's a half hour later.

Their coffee meeting unnerved her. Her friend had an air of male self-assurance about him that made her immediately uneasy yet at the same time thrilled her. They talked for over an hour, a guilty hour for Dr. Brittain because she wanted badly to keep talking, to arrange to meet her friend/patient again. She wanted to flirt, be involved with him. Since that meeting, she'd been having erotic fantasies in which they were married.

In one fantasy, they had a weekend ritual in which she slept in, and he, an early riser, drank coffee and read the newspaper downstairs. As she imagined it, one Saturday morning, he was in the kitchen making coffee, and she came downstairs unexpectedly. Naked, her hands bashfully covering her breasts, she breathlessly said, "I'm being a naughty girl. Instead of sleeping in, I've come down to interfere with your private time. I'm so bad!" She fluttered her eyelashes in mock remorse. In her fantasy, he took her over his knee and said, "You are a bad, bad girl." Then he playfully bit her bottom, gave her a mock spanking, and tickled her feet. And growled and teased. And made wild love with her in a big easy chair. Dr. Brittain couldn't stop thinking about this scenario, indulging her delicious daydreams. Were the daydreams to be fulfilled, she imagined she would be sublimely happy.

Reading between the lines, you may be able to sense that I was on her side, that I wished for her to have this womanly happiness, get rid of her dud husband and go for (what I thought was) a better life. She also imagined a scene with her real-life husband that had the same beginning but ended with her husband wimping out, unable to have sexual fun and join in on real lovemaking. I liked that variation too, the subplot in which her dud husband got his comeuppance. And after Dr. Brittain had told me about some of her fantasies, she announced that getting them off her chest had made her feel much better, and she thanked me. I had hardly said a word.

A few weeks later, Dr. Brittain's husband phoned and asked to see me. In our meeting, he told me his wife had gone to her parents' home and he didn't know whether she was coming back. He too wanted only to get his story off his chest, and I heard from neither him nor his wife again. I had hardly spoken to either of them, but my curt questions, my psychiatric demeanour, and the power of my cultural role were all that was needed.

Even though I had a hunch she wouldn't, I hoped Dr. Brittain would find sublime happiness. I'm a romantic, and I wanted her, a decent young woman who'd had bad luck and made a bad marriage, to discover a dreamy paradise. But such hopes were also my moment for caution: I'm suspicious of the sublime, especially since I was playing and enjoying the same game as my patient, agreeing with her delicious hopes and dreams. In Dr. Brittain's case, I was worried about something, part of her history I failed to draw to her attention, part of her history I didn't want to challenge: Why had she married a man with whom the dance of love and sex was so ungainly? She had eyes to see and a brain to think, and the evidence must have been there, don't you think? Or should I instead be saying that it was me, that *I* have eyes to see and a brain to think and the evidence was there for me too, don't you think? But the evidence was slight. She and I had had little time to talk about her life—her family, her sexual history, a collection of analogies that might have helped make sense of what was going on.

2

Show and Tell

Wise is the man who is content with the spectacle of life.
JOSÉ SARAMAGO, recipient of the Nobel Prize in Literature, 1998

IT'S NEW YEAR'S Day, 2014, and I'm in the state of Chiapas in Mexico, sitting on a bench in the Zócalo of San Cristóbal de las Casas watching the goings-on. As the scene unfolds, I'm typing what I see into my laptop—that is, I'm typing my *interpretation* of what I see into my laptop.

All the faces are brown, and although some people are in traditional Mayan dress, today many are wearing Western clothes, probably because it's a holiday. They are celebrating, dressed to kill, a New Year's version of the Easter parade that happens on the boardwalk out at The Beach in Toronto. Because I can't stop watching people, I'm aware that everyone is firing off clues to who they are: signals, language, expressions, glances, gestures. A nice couple is seated on a bench in front of me. He looks sixty but is probably forty-five. He has iron-grey hair and an imposing moustache the same colour, a Sunday shirt, and ragged jeans (because Mayan men are beardless, his moustache betrays mixed blood). His face is glum. Beside him is his wife—she has a wedding ring—who looks a few years younger. She is leaning her head against his shoulder and chattering happily, a lovely smile on her face. She's speaking Mayan, funny clicking sounds—*Quetzalcóatl, Tlaloc, tlamacazqui*—that I'll try to imitate once I move on. (I've tried to make the sounds before, so I know I won't succeed, but I'll still enjoy the attempt.) Once in a while she gets her husband to look down at her, even to smile back. She's wearing makeup, and the skin of her face is gorgeously smooth, a hint of rosiness in her lips and possibly a bit of extra colour on her cheeks. She's chunky and square like many Mayans, a bit on the plump side. Her ankles are weather-beaten, browner than the rest of her, the skin coarsened by the sun. But she has on black toenail polish.

I'm in love.

I'm happy too. I love this town and love watching the people. When I'm here, I don't have to worry about poor people because here everyone is poor, and they have the same fun I do. The girls are girlish and pink, the boys are noisy and full of mischief, and the grownups are disciplining their children and chattering away. I always romanticize such scenes when I'm in San Cristobal. When I was here fifty years ago, a *paseo* occurred every evening—young girls strolled demurely with their chaperones (mothers? aunts?) in a circle around the Zócalo while teenaged boys walked in the opposite direction alone or with their pals. The young men spoke only to the chaperones, never to the girls themselves. I was told that if a boy made a good impression on a chaperone, he might be invited to walk with them. When I'm here, I don't have to feel guilty about my well-off circumstances in Toronto.

My Mayan lady has a blanket—all the women carry blankets in which they keep possessions, including babies—and she occasionally holds it up to keep the sun off her face. She doesn't want her skin any darker, I guess. The blanket is store-bought and looks inexpensive, made of shiny synthetic material, and I can see the fold marks on it as if it's just been removed from the box where it's been waiting for this special day. Strange that she's chosen such a blanket; Mayans make and use colourful blankets and sell them everywhere. Maybe the blanket she's carrying seems modern or exotic to her, just as Mayan blankets are exotic to me. And now, she and her husband get up and walk away. She's wearing jeans with flowery patterns of glittery stuff on the bum, the same kind of glitter as on her sandals. She hangs on to her husband's arm, leaning into him, still chattering. He looks over at her, and I can see that he thinks she's terrific, adores her, but doesn't want to let on.

Oh dear. A handicapped woman is walking by with her husband and three children. She limps heavily, but that hasn't stopped her from getting dressed up. She knows she has nice legs because she's wearing black leggings (she's Mayan, so her legs aren't long) and a miniskirt that I can barely see below her jacket. Best of all, she has on a brilliant pair of high heels—patent leather, brand new. Wow! What nerve. Crippled, and walking in those things on the rough cobblestones. Eventually, she sits, and her husband and the two younger children walk on. Her oldest, a girl, stays with her, and once again there is a scene with a blanket. The daughter holds up the blanket in front of her mother—why? And suddenly I understand: she's not handicapped after all—her shoes are pinching her feet! Behind the blanket I catch glimpses of her putting bits of paper into the toe of one of her shoes—my God, are those heels ever high—trying to get her New Year's parade back on track. She is standard issue in San Cristóbal—boxy, but infatuated by her own wonders, her satisfaction with being who she is, a woman. Because she has her shoe off, I can see her foot: her toenails too are painted.

Thank God for nail polish in San Cristóbal de las Casas.

A boy of about nineteen walks by with a guitar over his shoulder. His jeans hang down on top of his runners exactly as they should. They also hang on his hips exactly as they should. His nondescript shirt looks perfect. And he strides along gracefully, proud, as he should be, that he's in his prime. If I hadn't lost my heart to the chattering lady with rosy lips and rosy cheeks, I'd definitely go for him. Alas, alas.

THIS IS A DESCRIPTION, not as good as George Eliot would have written, but my best try. Description is vitally important for the psychiatrist because it immunizes her just a little against misleading theories; sticking to description guarantees she won't say her patient's unusual behaviour is caused by his genes or by a disease—determinism—and won't say her patient behaves in an unusual way because he chooses to act that way—free will. To the psychiatrist, determinism and free will are theories that, in this scene (and in the psychiatrist's office), are not only useless, but seriously misleading. The pathetic philosophers who raise this question think there's a competition—but there isn't. No one will win because free will and determinism inhabit different logical universes, can't compete because they aren't on the same playing field. I've described the scene on the Zócalo using a language that suits my mood, picking words, phrases, and details that will influence you: I'm persuading you that the scene is wonderful. It's another theory, of course, seen through the distorting glasses I put on when I visit remote communities.

So why have I begun with this? If I can get you to become my psychiatrist for a few minutes, and if you stick to what I've described, you'll have to keep in mind that even though I've been faithfully descriptive, you've still heard only my *interpretation* of the events on the Zócalo. In other words, the characters I've described turn out not to be the real focus; I've glamourized and romanticized the scene, and that's what you ought to notice. Since you are now the psychiatrist, your attention is on me, the person telling the story; I'm the only person about whom you can reach any conclusions. Since everything I say informs you about me—my topics, my style and tone, my focus, my commentary—the manner in which I told the story should tell you a lot. I'm assigning you the job of doing exactly what the psychiatrist does in her office. Since psychiatrists have no tests and don't do physical examinations, you have no other data. You're stuck with analyzing my speeches and my stories.

Among other things, you will have noticed that I'm rather jolly, and you'd be right (I'm jolly here and there, now and then, but I'm also crabby). This is a fact about me, a datum, a piece of raw material you can study. If a scientist studies the brain, she's also looking for data, but not at all like the things you can figure out about me—me as distinct from my brain. The objective study of the brain produces neurophysiological—not psychiatric—knowledge. Unlike the behavioural trait called jolliness, you can get hold of a brain. It's an organ that can be studied objectively and scientifically. Rather than doing human things, the brain generates electrical fields, metabolizes glucose, manufactures and breaks down transmitters—all things that can be studied biologically. A brain also has mass, texture, colour, temperature, and a system of blood circulation, and as you study it, there's no person in sight. The more you study it, the more a brain resembles a blob of neurons firing off electrical impulses—an organ, all right, but only one part of a person. If you pee on my kitchen floor, it's you who did it, not your brain. And if you lust after the handsome devil you've just met, it's you who is full of lust, not your brain.

It turns out that jolliness is too complicated to be understood by studying the brain, so you'll have to tackle it by using another discipline: psychology/psychiatry. Then you can say things like, "As opposed to being located in the brain, the location of jolliness is in Gordon Warme, a person." The manoeuvre of switching disciplines when a problem gets too complicated is common. If a particle physicist can't explain magnification because the particle behaviours involved in magnification are too complicated, she passes the problem on to someone from a different discipline: optics. If a cellular physiologist can't figure out how to stop the growth of a cancer cell, she passes the problem over to a surgeon who cuts the tumour out. If I want to eat meat, I don't study the disciplines of animal husbandry and the food chain, I rely on the discipline of marketing, go across the street, and buy a pork chop. When our philosophical musings fail to surrender the meaning of life, we switch to religion and other superstitions: health foods, scientism, political correctness. Carl Sagan summed this up by saying, "If you want to make an apple pie from scratch, you must first create the universe."

It may be possible to find activities in the brain that correlate with my jolliness, but surprisingly, if I *pretend* to be in a jolly mood, you'll likely find the same brain activity as if I'm genuinely jolly. Since I have a brain, but I am not a brain, I see myself doing the same things I see other people do: hoping, sinning, philandering, arguing, grieving, celebrating. And as for the intangible gadget in my head that I call my mind, it isn't separate from me at all. It doesn't even exist. *Mind* is just a made-up word to summarize my thinking and my performances including things like hoping, sinning, philandering, arguing, grieving, and celebrating.

To be a reader, you must have an interest in the topic I'm writing about; were I a travel writer, for example, you'd concentrate on what I've said about San Cristóbal and the Mayan people. To a lesser extent, you'd be interested in me, the person who is writing. As a psychiatrist, it's the other way around; you are less interested in my topics and more interested in me and why I write and speak the way I do. So, for now, you are the psychiatrist, gleaning from my stories whatever you can.

But none of the things you figure out will be solid facts. My jolliness, for example, isn't an essential truth about me. Apart from what you see on the surface, there are many ways of talking about my jolliness. Among other things, you may suspect that I'm secretly aware of its manipulative effects, even if I insist to you that jolliness is just the way I am, who I am, what I am. "Don't be ridiculous," I might answer. "I've always been like that. When I was a kid I was like that." Never mind my disclaimers. When you are my shrink, you mustn't take my words at face value; you must insist that there are more ways of talking about good cheer than are immediately apparent. It's perfectly possible that my jollity aims to disarm you, or it might serve to patch over an inner sadness of mine, or whatever else you can figure out that it might mean. So let me lie down on your couch and free associate, tell you more, and more, and more.

I wrote the Zócalo story as an email to my children and my grandchildren, letting them know I'm having a good time here in Mexico. I'm trying to impress them, make them love good old me, their Opa. My children and grandchildren know I weep at movies and at the Santa Claus parade, so none of this will surprise them, but there's no harm underlining for them how sensitive and fine a person I am. A worthier aim would be if I wrote the email because I want to inspire my children and grandchildren so that in future when they travel, they'll look closely at things, therefore have more fun. By being amateur anthropologists, they might also be better people. And maybe, just maybe, I knew I'd put the story into this book so I could impress you, my psychiatrist.

I'm here in San Cristóbal for another reason that just popped into my mind. (This is amazing, Doc! I have to admit that lying here on your couch frees up my thinking.) I realize I'm reassuring myself that when my father was far away—I didn't know where—for three years during World War II, he was okay, just as today I can see that these Mayans, also far away, are similarly okay. And since my family was an immigrant family, a minority, I can see by watching the Mayan minority group that minorities are just fine; I'm reassuring myself that the poor people of Chiapas have as good a life as I do. But that's still not the whole story because I'm also here to have fun, an adventure. What I've told you is not scientific information; it's just thoughts that have welled up in my mind that alert me to new sides of myself, ready to be shoved aside by other thoughts that may occur to me as I lie here on your psychiatric couch. So now you know more, that I am sentimental, vain, jolly, concerned, and a bit bruised by my history.

When I speculate this way about what I've seen and how to understand it, it's called insight; in Socrates's *agora*, it was called the examined life, the only one worth living. Above the oracle at Delphi is inscribed *Gnothi se auton*, usually translated as "Know thyself." But Socrates says there's a better translation: "Look at thyself." The command insists that we should be artists of self-watching. Each artist watches in his own way, just as I, half artist, study patients in my own way. In the consulting room, I'm lost in my thoughts, watching from an odd, nonexistent vantage point, baffled and fascinated by what I see. I am a pondering fool, a fanatic of observation and sparse comment.

The understanding comes from seeing connections, analogies, and repetitions. And it's not just *seeing* connections, it's also being *shown* connections, having connections described to me. That's where you (don't forget that you're now my psychiatrist) come into the story. You are the extra observer who sees new things, attends closely as I speculate out loud about my New Year's Day in San Cristóbal, and points out things I haven't noticed. My *conscious* reason for describing the rosy-cheeked lady, the proud but hobbling woman who rivalled her in fashion, and the confident young man with the guitar, is to get you thinking about description, how pervasive it is, and how easy it is to think that, in revealing my fantasies about things that are far away and about minority groups, I am explaining those fantasies, when actually I'm not. I'm just describing them. But you may have other ideas, may have noticed there are things I neglected to describe.

Is there a touch of smugness in the way I talk about these things? If you are my psychiatrist, you mustn't just tell me I'm smug because I'd be annoyed and wouldn't take you seriously. So what will you do? Well, you'll have to be clever. Ideally, you'll come up with an odd way of approaching the topic of smugness, a tiny little perturbation, but my mind is blank, so I have no tips for you right now. In any case, keep my smugness in the back of your mind and hope that a bright idea comes along. Maybe something I say will strike you as being related and will suggest a way of drawing my smugness to my attention.

MANY WANT BIOLOGICAL explanations for everything people do, but obviously, that won't work in describing my reaction—I'm still the patient in this scenario—to the scene on the Zócalo of San Cristóbal. When biology can't be nailed down, most of us accept what some consider a second-best option: speculation. I've tried not to do that, to simply do show and tell, give descriptions, what kindergarten children do every morning in school. Even that isn't quite right because I've really only told stories, given off a cluster of signals—symbols—that convey to you my ways of seeing the world, delivering messages about how I want to be understood, messages neither good nor bad but important to me and decipherable by you or by whoever else sees the prompts I'm giving off. Amazingly, even though psychiatrists do show and tell all the time, and even though it's obvious that all of us see the world through eyeglasses that we've each designed differently, many colleagues haven't figured this out. When it's said that psychiatric patients have biological disorders, it's the wildest of speculations, appropriate neither as science nor as literature, and not up to the standard expected of an elementary school student.

A woman in my building got on the elevator with her four-year-old granddaughter. I said to the woman in a teasing voice, "I see you're taking your doggie for a walk." The little girl smiled, then looked up at her grandmother and said, "Woof!" (Ooh! My heart aches at the memory. Now I'm in love with that little girl.) We humans are preternaturally skilled at connecting things, at having one thing stand in for another, and at finding resemblances. That's why we can talk, write, and read. We're so good at this that often we don't need to be shown what's going on. A child figures out early on that she can cuddle a stick and pretend it's a baby. And if another child sees this symbolic act, she immediately understands what's going on. (Chimpanzees too can cuddle a stick and pretend it's a baby, but this act of representation can't be shared with another chimpanzee. A human can see what the chimp is up to, but another chimp cannot.) Speech, writing, ideograms, and hieroglyphics stand for words, ideas, and things, and all are examples of this amazing human capacity. If one thing stands in for another, I can expand my list to include toys, photographs, dreams, thoughts, art, miniatures, all re-creations. Trading, selling, buying, markets—all demand that one thing should stand in for another: coins, goods, trinkets, favours, money, sex. Add to the list robots, automatons, masks, disguises, and Halloween. Joe DiMaggio arranged that six red roses be delivered to Marilyn Monroe's grave twice a week for twenty years: the roses stand in for love—and make me choke up, just a little bit. (Are you, my psychiatrist, still there? Did my phrase "choke up" catch your attention? When I described the scene on the Zócalo, I was also a bit choked up. If you're doing your job you'll have noticed—and this may be a good time to point it out to me—that I overdo it, have a small habit of choking up. This mushiness of mine and my romantic tendencies may be worth paying attention to.)

The important mirror neurons in the brain are involved in this repeating and re-creating, but you and I are still the ones who are spellbound and enthralled by pictures, electric trains, and dollhouses. And isn't it great to think that you may once have been in love like Joe DiMaggio? An infant, early on, imitates: open your mouth and he opens his mouth, smile and he smiles, frown and he frowns. I love watching this in fourteen-month-old children who, given simple pictures of everyday objects, even schematic outlines, open their eyes in astonishment and name things: "cup," "car," "shoe," and for a dog, "woof." Of course, the child who names things is doing what I did when I wrote about the Zócalo. He is not explaining; rather, he is *showing* you what he sees, describing and identifying it.

3
The Awkward Secret

Tell all the truth but tell it slant—
Success in circuit lies . . .
Too bright for our infirm Delight
The Truth's superb surprise.
EMILY DICKINSON

I HAVE BITTER MEDICINE for you. The story of the Zócalo of San Cristóbal was the bit of sugar that helps the medicine go down, that sugar-jolliness of mine. As my psychiatrist, you'll have made a quick interpretation of what you heard me say—your initial description—and then, by looking beyond that first description, you'll have interpreted the scene again—and again and again. You will have *re*described things. These later versions of what I said will cast a different light on what I thought I was doing, will have changed things just a bit. Emily Dickinson's aphorism above alerts you to my slyness, that I am actually talking about the confusing, profound, and controversial advice of Ludwig Wittgenstein: "Philosophy is a battle against the bewitchment of our intelligence by means of language."

I have to dose you with bitter medicine because you psychiatrists are making a mess of things. Although you probably don't know it, your errors lead to discrimination and bigotry, the attitude that we mental patients are inferior to you. (As you can see, I'm a difficult patient, pushy, and opinionated. Are you irked, starting to think of me as noncompliant? Or have you come up with something less insulting than the word *noncompliant*? You'll be relieved to know we can stop our patient-psychiatrist game at the end of the next paragraph.)

In any case, I'm out to unsettle you, determined to get you thinking, or better, get you to *change* your thinking. I'm talking about your blindness, the blindness of psychiatrists who don't want to know the obvious. Your psychiatric expertise is, I'm saying, limited to perspectivism, which means that when you notice something about me, you notice it from a certain point of view, and that there are countless other angles from which I could have been studied. The same goes for me. Being limited to showing me there are more angles on what I, your patient, have told you about the Zócalo may seem to a doctor to be a weak way of operating, mainly because it doesn't seem to be a treatment. It also won't lead you to a diagnosis. Mostly, you'll only be able to come up with a bunch of connections and parallels—varieties of interpretation. What's also hard is to realize that no such thing exists as psychiatric explanation, explanation being the aim of science but not of psychiatry. Because you psychiatrists have no hard evidence, psychiatric explanation is impossible.

If you ask me why I think free speech is a good thing, I'll reply, "It's my preference, my taste, that free speech is a good thing. There's no rationalizing these things, no explaining them scientifically. It's the way a nice liberal—I'm less liberal than I let on—thinks the world ought to be. Nor can anyone explain why I think hurting others without cause is a bad thing, or why others think hurting someone is fun or a sexual turn-on—although metaphysicians and meta-psychologists,[1] those who believe in essences and hidden, underlying facts, may disagree.

At a dinner party, I was placed beside a woman, charming and a perfect match for my social pretensions, interests, and habits. As the host intended, we talked up a storm and later went out once or twice.

---

1 *Metadata* is often called data about data or information about information. Correspondingly, *metaphysics* is information about the topic of physics, not about the theories of physics. *Meta-psychology* is information about the topic of psychology in general, not about the theories of psychology. A metaphysician isn't doing physics, nor is a meta-psychologist doing psychology. They are talking *about* these subjects.

A few weeks later, my friend, the host, phoned. "What happened with you and Sarah?"

I mumbled something vague.

"Aha," he said. "No 'click' factor."

Yes, the click factor. How does a scientist explain *that*? If she tried, she'd also have to explain why Sarah, although she didn't click with me, will certainly click with someone else, someone who, as soon as he sees her, will feel a connection, be smitten. I haven't the slightest doubt that Sarah will ignite the mind of some lucky fellow, that he will experience a *coup de foudre*. When I think back, I'm baffled that Sarah didn't click for me, fear that I must have made a mistake, wonder whether the non-existent click was actually a click and I didn't notice.

The scientist, in principle, cannot explain such events. Why not? Among other reasons, it's because that datum, that human event, that magic moment that someone wants to explain is a one-time thing, unique to the particular man and the particular woman involved. There's no chance that anything like that could ever be predicted or replicated. Besides, it isn't a single *datum*. Clicks and enthrallments and human shenanigans involve so many factors, millions of them, that even the plural form, *data*, is far too weak. And there's no chance that anything a crazy or neurotic person does could ever be predicted or replicated either, because craziness, like falling in love, is a unique event or, better, a unique *performance*, and performances are not what science studies. But if I talk to you about what happened with Sarah, and even if I can't explain it, you'll understand by way of personal analogies, parallels, and connections. "Oh, I see," you'll say. "No click factor," "No chemistry," "You didn't hit it off," "She wasn't your type," or, as I once joked with a patient: "I see what you mean, Mr. Brownlee. She was too fat, too thin, too tall, too short, too old, too young, the wrong religion." Only a series of analogies captures what did, didn't, or could have happened.

Part of the confusion is because, in ordinary life, we say *explain* when we only mean we understand something in human terms. The speculative comments made by sports broadcasters ("he choked once he got to the Wimbledon final"; "she's always been intimidated by Maria Sharapova"; "beating Serena Williams gave her back her confidence") are common ways of understanding why people act as they do, except that when the psychiatrist tries to explain, she struggles to avoid standard formulas and platitudes. With most patients, the psychiatrist tries to say what's never been said before.

In my day-to-day life I'm liable to explain why a politician resorts to clichés, talking points, and sound bites by saying he's an ass, a coward, or an idiot. But these are not explanations. All I'm doing is describing him using the silly and insulting metaphors that I like to apply to such people. I'm certainly not giving a scientific explanation of his behaviour.

One of the psychiatrist's awkward secrets is that, in a sense, what she does is ordinary. She does only one thing: using the currently fashionable form of psychological speculation, she talks with her patients. The ghosts of Vladimir Nabokov and Thomas Szasz, famous enemies of psychiatry, will now squirm in ecstasy at the thought that psychiatry is a lot of hot air. But these ecstatics are wrong because the psychiatric doctor has something up her sleeve, and it's not highbrow language, fancy ideas, or an extraordinary talent for plain talk. It's that she absolutely always "listens with the third ear"—that is to say, she takes a metapsychological attitude toward everything she hears.[2]

Here is Shakespeare in *Love's Labour's Lost*, showing us a metapsychological comment made by Rosaline in response to what Berowne says to her:

> *Berowne*: And, to begin: wench, so God help me, law!
> My love to thee is sound, *sans* crack or flaw.
> *Rosaline*: *Sans "sans,"* I pray you. (5.2.414–416)

Instead of making a comment *in response* to Berowne's declaration—"I don't think we're a good match, Berowne" or "Yes, and perhaps we should go out to dinner sometime," Rosaline stands back and notices the *style* of Berowne's statement, and makes a (rude) comment *about* what he said; she has listened with the third ear and responded

---

2 I don't mean *metapsychology* as psychoanalysts use the word: their reference is to the ego, the id, the superego, drives, cathexes, and internal objects, the imaginary mental "structures" or "things" I think psychoanalysts should forget about. Their word *metapsychology* has no hyphen.

with a meta-comment that I would paraphrase as, "It's stupid to use that phony French word *sans*." When the psychiatrist comments meta-psychologically (she's never rude like Rosaline), she is reclassifying what her patient is saying. Instead of responding to her patient's words in the ordinary way, she makes comments about her patient's *style* of speaking. Of course, this reclassifying business appears in all conversation, although rarely as explicitly and with such single-minded intent as when the psychiatrist does it in her office. Instead of plain talk, saying, "Wow, you got tickets for the Madonna concert," anyone might instead give a meta-psychological response, "How the devil did you manage to get tickets to see Madonna?" Or, when told by a friend how handsome George Clooney is, instead of saying, "Yeah, he's a pretty handsome guy," we might, like a psychiatrist, say, "Don't you think you're going overboard about how handsome George Clooney is?"—again, a meta-psychological statement. The differences between what we all do in conversations and what psychiatrists (at least the well-trained ones) do are threefold:

1. The psychiatrist begins the appointment/conversation with a noncommittal greeting, which, except for the "noncommittal" part, is ordinary, everyday behaviour.

2. After that, she listens exclusively with the third ear and, as the appointment progresses and depending on what she hears, makes only meta-comments. Instead of chatting, answering questions, giving advice, or offering support, she makes comments *about* the patient's wish to chat, *about* his questions, *about* his wishes for advice, and *about* speeches or behaviours that suggest the patient needs support.

3. After a predetermined time, the psychiatrist stops listening with the third ear, reverts to ordinary talk, and announces that the time is up. If necessary, she then discusses business matters (money, appointment changes) and says goodbye.

I'm guessing that your reaction to this set of rules will be a meta-comment, an observation about me, assessing me psychologically: "It looks to me, Warme, as though you're an old-fashioned Freudian."

Since this is not a treatise on how to conduct a psychiatric interview, I won't defend my guidelines but ask instead that you notice that you have listened to me with the third ear. Instead of *responding* to what I said ("Oh, really? Why does the psychiatrist do it that way?"), you have made a comment *about* what I said ("Hmm, I see that you're a Freudian!"). That the psychiatrist sticks to the meta position puzzles patients for the first few minutes of an initial appointment, but most are quickly intrigued by their psychiatrist's focus on their psychological style, mainly because they immediately start learning things about themselves. A few patients don't like it, want to gab and be hearty and want the same kind of hearty response from the psychiatrist. Contrariwise, some patients are determined to speak only about unhappiness and want from the psychiatrist only a series of sympathetic responses, uninterested in comments *about* their typical way of talking.

Another example: I might say to a patient, "Another way of talking about your wonderful mother would be to say that it's important for you to *convince* me that you have a wonderful mother." This metapsychological comment undermines what my patient has been saying, not because his story is wrong but because every story can be told many ways. It's not the truth, or a fact, or more basic than how the patient first told the story. It's only another angle on things. In some cases, such a psychiatric nudge leads nowhere; in other cases it leads to extreme new perspectives on how the patient thinks: "If I didn't praise the bitch, I'd have to kill her," or more typically, "Convince you? Hmm. I never noticed that. What are you driving at? Do you mean I might not admire her as much as I say? Well, I guess sometimes I . . ." Any one of us might say that anger at his mother "causes" this patient to do the opposite, to praise her, but we'd only be doing ordinary psychological talk—it would not be a scientific/explanatory statement.

Around the dinner table, there's no need to worry about such ordinary chatter. "She's rebelling," we might say. "Her parents totally screwed her up by being so moralistic and sticking their noses into everything she did." I'll give more examples of such psychiatric talk in later chapters. But whether it's gossip or the careful and unusual version of such talk used by the psychiatrist, it doesn't explain scientifically because it's really description and redescription, analogous to my description of the people on the Zócalo of San Cristóbal de las Casas: the rosy woman who smiled so lovingly at her husband, the hobbling woman who wore the patent-leather high-heeled shoes that pinched, and the young man who walked so proudly carrying his guitar. Talk about a rebellious girl whose behaviour is "explained" by saying she had intrusive, moralistic parents is nothing more than a description of thoughts and imaginings any of us might have. We might agree and we might be right, but only in the sense that that's how we, individually and in this culture, tend to think about these things. It's not a causal or etiological explanation, and therefore not scientific. But it might be medical—as long as we don't insist that everything "medical" has to be scientific.

MENTAL PATIENTS DO strange things, occasionally offensive things, but so do those of us who don't carry the stigma of being "mental cases." Just the same, most of us are quick to judge: someone is healthy (better, ordinary, conventional), and someone else is sick (weird, weak, inferior), statements based on false explanations: because they have abnormalities—*so-called* abnormalities—the mad and the sad are victims of a disease. I disagree. I say that the mad and the sad are members of a social subgroup, well known in every culture, whose members, rather than presenting themselves as standard issue, present themselves as unconventional, bizarre, tragic, or weird.

Trying or forcing a cultural subgroup to change against its will is cultural genocide, and in the case of pedophiles, systematic killers, and drunk drivers, most of us would agree that suppressing such categories of cultural life is right and proper. But the mad, most of whom are harmless, don't strike me as having a way of life that must be suppressed. Their behaviour may be troubling to you or me, but that's not reason enough. Just because some of the mad commit more crimes than the rest of us doesn't mean we have the right to confine other mad people against their wills if no crime has been committed; because more men than women commit murders doesn't lead to the ridiculous conclusion that all men should be jailed, confined against their will. Statistics can be misused—*are* misused.

The subgroup of people called the mentally ill defends itself poorly and is therefore not listened to tolerantly, probably because its members present themselves in preposterous or nonstandard ways. My naïve colleagues ought finally to be put under pressure to stop treating psychiatric patients as offenders—finally, because the mistreatment of crazy people has gone on since time immemorial. That nowadays hospital lockups are spiffy and expensive hides the awfulness of what goes on: forcing or manipulating patients into taking drugs, undergoing electric shocks, and worst of all, ruling that they are biologically abnormal. In the end, this means permanent stigmatization as inferior human beings.

The psychiatrists who most need to smarten up are those who currently hold positions in universities. They are amazingly blind—although not as blind as you may think. Since I am one of them, I can tell you that when I clap them on the shoulder in the corridors of the Centre for Addiction and Mental Health, the hospital where I work, and tease them about their biological "findings," they don't argue with me. Nor do they argue when I remind them that sugar pills help depressed people almost as well as antidepressants. This shouldn't surprise anyone: part of the definition of severe depression and what distinguishes it from other forms of psychosis is that those who suffer from it have spontaneous remissions; that is to say, they usually get better on their own.

I'm not suggesting utopia will be born. Nonsense will always be with us. Fervent belief in psychoanalysis lasted seventy to eighty years. Don't get me wrong; I've learned plenty from studying Freud and from being in psychoanalysis myself, but to the extent that psychoanalysis defines patients as damaged or diseased, it has taken the same villainous turn as biological psychiatry. Medical fashions—yes, these bad habits are fashions—change slowly. But just the same, we ought to goad psychiatrists, shame them into waking up, shame *me* into waking up, and maybe you too.

In their own way, talking doctors are as useless as biological psychiatrists. If the only thing in play is description—mere description—how can anything worthwhile happen in the psychiatrist's office? The patient describes what's on his mind and the psychiatrist describes what's on *her* mind. But the talking doctor has something up her sleeve; she isn't a beginner. She's a journeyman, a performer, a connecter, skilled at finding analogies and antonyms; rather than chatting, she wants to be a meta-psychological supplement, a helpful nuisance (*nuisance* is a euphemism; what I mean is that she is a stinging gadfly, a seductive Mephistopheles) who reclassifies everything she hears, including pointing out to her patient his darkness. She speaks of him meta-venereally, meta-sinfully, and worst crime of all, meta-gloriously—his sin of pride. The psychiatrist consistently stands back and attends to what she hears with her third ear, then *shows* her patient what she has heard, especially those things she's heard that others don't want to admit they've heard. She shows, and shows, and shows, thus shedding light on what her patient is doing, expanding his awareness of his own life, especially because her descriptions, rather than being singular, are plural: she repeatedly *re*describes what's going on, making analogies and parallels and variations on those analogies and parallels.

If you are the patient, she'll keep *showing* you what you are doing and saying, and once she's done, you won't be cured but you'll know yourself better. Therefore, like her, I'll *show* you something, this time about ambiguity—four ambiguity stories.

1. It's strange that my waste, my poop, doesn't smell bad to me, yet everyone else's poop smells terrible. It can't be simple learning because I'm sure that my parents, like all parents, trained me to be offended by my poop: "Oh, *phew! Ugh!* Did you go poo-poo? Is your diaper full? Let's get rid of this awful poopy diaper," all said with grimaces and giggles about the horrible mess being cleaned up. Were I simply to have learned from my parents' words, I'd hate the smell of my bowel movements—but the truth is that I'm not much bothered by them (I can confess this because I know that you aren't much bothered by the smell of yours either). But don't ask me to touch my bowel movements; I can do it, but I don't want to. Therefore, I must have figured out that certain important things are to be reacted to ambiguously—the smell of my bowel movements isn't too bad, sort of interesting, but the touch would be hideous, and the same substance produced by you is horrible on all counts. (I've had a couple of ordinary patients who shamefacedly confessed that they didn't mind the smell of their spouse's poop, and there's also the example of coprophilia, those with a high interest in excretory products, people who sometimes eat them or require them for sexual arousal, but these are extreme cases.)

2. I'm now in Puerto Escondido, Mexico, collecting examples that will illustrate the points I'm making. It's hot, thirty-three degrees Celsius, and I've just walked to the market and back, which took three hours (I got lost). After such a long walk in the midday sun, I'm more than damp, so if the attractive woman here on the roof of the Hotel Flor de Maria decides I'm old, she'll say to herself that I smell; if she decides that I'm well preserved for my age, she'll say that I reek of maleness—the ambiguity is whether my smell is sexy or offensive.

3. It's an hour later. I said *hola* to the woman when I sat down, and we've had a conversation. She's about fifty and has a mass of greying hair, big waves flowing over the sides of her face and neck. Because it's hot, her hair must be a nuisance, sweaty too. I've barely met her, but the woman (I never did catch her name) punctuates our conversation with pats on my arm, flashes of her eyes, and cheery chuckles. It's not me; I saw her doing this with a man at her table in the dining room last night. But maybe, just maybe, she thinks that I reek of maleness. I like her, especially when I complain of my age and she says, "Like fine wine, better with age." (Pat, pat.) As we talk, I'm surprised to realize that she is smart. What's going on? Aren't giggly, histrionic women supposed to be airheads? Aren't all women airheads? How come she is two opposite things at once, both a bit of a ditz and smart as a whip? Hasn't she been properly raised, to think of herself as a nitwit? She's American, but knows all about how the Canadian parliamentary system works, very different from the American presidential system. Jayne Mansfield, a professionally trained airhead, is said to have had the highest IQ on record, spoke five languages, and was a classically trained pianist and violinist. Mansfield's comment: Her public was "more interested in 40-21-35."

4. As I walk on the beach here in Puerto Escondido, I am assailed by ideas for this book, and my imagination is transformed by trivial sights into episodes, examples, introductions. If I don't take my walk, I start trying to explain things, as influenced by our technological, progress-oriented culture as anyone else. Because I'm a doctor and want to explain things, my stories can be boring; in thrall to

imaginativeness, I do better. What's the point I'm making? It's that the first three sentences of this point define me as passive—"I am assailed by ideas," "my imagination is transformed by trivial sights," and I am "influenced by our... culture," and I am "in thrall to imaginativeness." Ordinarily I'm determined that we're best off if we *don't* think of ourselves as passive, and instead describe ourselves as the agents of our own actions and ways of life. In the meantime, my lady friend, also the agent of her own life, has abandoned me and is now sitting on the other side of the rooftop terrace waiting for her Spanish tutor.

Second, those sentences illustrate my current point, the ubiquity and importance of ambiguity. Of course I am not "assailed *by* ideas," nor am I "victimized *by* my culture," yet all the same the ideas *do* come upon me unbidden, and I *am* a victim of my culture, although I'm really not, even when I am. And since the behaviour of the mad and tragic people in my office is equally ambiguous, psychiatrists must surrender claims of scientific explanation, which doesn't allow for ambiguity.

Why the devil would we humans operate this way? Wouldn't logical propositions get us further? The easy answer is that a mechanistic world would be boring, as most would agree. But the important reason is that ambiguity gets us doing the thing that makes us such a successful species—thinking. That's why the psychiatrist talks so little: faced by silence, her patient struggles, tries to figure out what his doctor wants, and eventually figures out for himself what he ought to talk about. Whether for good or bad, ambiguity and quietness are the precipitants, the incitements, and the occasions of creativity, uniqueness, and genius. It's worth noticing that, as I talk about ambiguity, I'm *showing* you things, giving examples and descriptions of things.

Having thought things over, should you cut the Gordian knot, fix things once and for all, and finish with dithering? Or should you consult with the oracle at Delphi, the most important source of wisdom, receive from it the precious information delivered only by the Pythia, the strange, psychotic women who dispense ambiguous prophesies?

PART TWO

BIOLOGY ON THE COUCH

4

Opinion versus Evidence

Pisces mortui solum cum flumine natant
(Only dead fish go with the flow).
ANONYMOUS

DR. KAYOKO KIFUJI mishandled things, and her patient, Rebecca Riley, paid the price. Dr. Kifuji has also paid a price, but she didn't lose her licence to practise medicine, nor did her colleagues rebuke her. Tufts Medical Center in Boston defended her, and their spokesperson told the TV show *60 Minutes* that "the care we provided was appropriate and within responsible professional standards."

> When Rebecca Riley was 28 months old, based primarily on the complaints of her mother that she was "hyper" and had difficulty sleeping, psychiatrist Kayoko Kifuji... diagnosed Rebecca with attention deficit hyperactivity disorder (ADHD). Kifuji prescribed clonidine, a [anti] hypertensive drug with significant sedating properties...
>
> By the time Rebecca was three years old... Kifuji had given Rebecca an additional diagnosis of bipolar disorder and prescribed... the antipsychotic Seroquel and the anticonvulsant Depakote.
>
> At the age of four, Rebecca was dead.
>
> At the time of her death, Rebecca had a life-threatening amount of clonidine—enough to kill her—in her body, according to the former director of the Massachusetts toxicology lab and the medical director

> of a regional poison control center. . . . Rebecca's abusive parents went to prison for the over-drugging that led to their daughter's death.[1]

Such tragedies happen because Dr. Kifuji acted on the basis of *opinion* rather than on the basis of *evidence*, an opinion that was dead wrong: she took the metaphor of disease to be a biological fact. The only thing that can be said on her behalf is that she acted according to a psychiatric fashion, a superstition that would have been jettisoned long ago had psychiatrists kept the scientific method in the mix. Since Dr. Kifuji had knowledge of no disease, she ought to have held her fire and realized that there was nothing biological that she could do. This particular superstition has led modern psychiatrists astray, steered them into doing what Dr. Kifuji did, to blindly giving powerful drugs that have no specific action except to subdue patients.

The opinion that psychiatric patients have biological abnormalities is actually a morality play, an insulting judgment, a hierarchy of worth that implies that psychiatric patients are biologically inferior to the rest of us, just as blacks, homosexuals, Jews, and women were once deemed inferior to white, straight, gentile males like me—deemed *biologically* inferior. When the problems are serious, psychiatrists all too often admit to their faith position, saying things like "There *must* be a biological disorder." This is as religious an opinion as the words to Schiller's *Ode to Joy*: "Somewhere over the starry vault there *must* be a loving father." Then, believing a cause exists, psychiatrists conclude that the problem must have a solution. When they resort to "solve problems" thinking (it's an excellent model for a surgeon, by the way) psychiatrists have latched onto a way of thinking that's pretty well useless in their line of work.

Such errors spring from the medical tendency to cling to Aristotelian logic, the stupendous underpinning for Newtonian physics with which we can build bridges, revolutionize industry, throw snowballs, and fight traditional wars. Correctly used, Aristotelian logic is also good for

1 Bruce E. Levine, "America's Mental Health Industry Is a Threat to Our Sanity," *Truthout* (January 2012). http://www.truth-out.org/7-reasons-americas-mental-health-industry-threat-our-sanity/1326036648.

diagnosing and treating most non-psychiatric medical disorders including cancer, diabetes, and pneumonia. Aristotle's logic is founded on the idea that the world comprises discrete things that have qualities. When doctors in every specialty except psychiatry use this logic—thinking of our patients as things that have qualities, that patients are bodies with diseases—this mindset works very well.

Three things have interfered with the habit of relying on Aristotelian logic across the board: first, the theory of relativity; second, quantum mechanics; third, the writings of twentieth-century philosophers like Ludwig Wittgenstein and Richard Rorty. These three movements interfere with the universal applicability of Aristotelian logic, and in psychiatry they interfere with the idea that people are bodies with diseases, objects with qualities. Because that logic doesn't work for human behaviour, we now do double-think: we recognize that there are many universes of discourse, each important in their proper area of applicability but useless in others. If you apply a form of logic in the wrong place you'll fail; you'll quickly find that if you try to use Newtonian physics—it's Aristotelian through and through—to romance the girl next door, you'll fail. Even if you use dozens of biological tests—brain scans, search out the light chains in her blood, her red and white blood cells, every test in the book—neither you nor she will have a handle on romance.

In contrast, when dealing with elementary particles or human behaviour, and when writing novels, we use another form of logic—interactional logic. In those instances, we understand the world as being made up of things *that are in articulation with other things*: people live embedded in language games with other people; time and space have powerful effects on each other, indeed, change each other; elementary particles like electrons and neutrons have instantaneous effects on each other, even when they are unimaginable distances apart. Furthermore, when we observe these particles—articulate with them—our acts of observation actually change the way the particles behave. The latter thinking works for psychiatrists and romancers, but Newtonian/Aristotelian philosophy—the idea of people being objects with qualities—does not.

Last week, for example, a student told me of her struggles with youngsters on an inpatient ward (she lives *in articulation* with the youngsters, I might have written), those said to have a disease called anorexia nervosa. When we doctors work with them, we are bewildered. We can't understand why these youngsters (more articulation, involvement) don't just eat something, why they are so desperate to be thin. Their refusal to eat is frightening—some die—their complaints of fatness preposterous, their skeletal appearance obvious. As the student described how some of her patients must be tube-fed, I remembered going through the same bewilderment with such patients forty years ago. Not only did I remember, I began to re-experience my frustration from years ago, began thinking in the language of solving problems. *There must be something we can do, damn it. After all these years, has nothing changed? Isn't this new generation of doctors smart enough to get into their patients' souls, the place in these young patients where they've gotten themselves screwed up? Are they twiddling their thumbs while these kids kill themselves?* You will have noticed that nothing in my descriptive questioning of events suggests that my student or the patients—or even I—are inert things that have qualities. Instead, I used language that denotes the interactions of human beings.

In the face of such tragedies, many psychiatrists resort to urgent measures, feel compelled to do something about an abnormal quality that they assume is inside the patient. Even though they have no clue what the abnormality is or how this invisible fiend might be got rid of, they still want to wipe it out—which is how Dr. Kifuji got herself in trouble. The drugs she prescribed do indeed subdue people, so families, patients, and doctors are sometimes satisfied on that ground, but more commonly families and patients hate the effects of the drugs. I don't prescribe such drugs; their horrible side effects, some of them permanent, are too much for me. In anticipation of something to which I will give a good deal of attention in chapter 16, I would add that the problematic method of solving problems ("do-something" thinking) is commoner in men. More valuable to the psychiatrist may be a type of thinking commoner in women, the acknowledgement that odd behaviour is a mystery (contemplative, artistic, and speculative thinking).

When given a prescription, patients are often satisfied because they've participated in a well-known social ritual, one of countless rituals that give relief to humans, the most culture-bound of creatures—

even if nothing substantial has happened. And, of course, participating in rituals is a good example of how humans *articulate* with one another. As a family doctor friend said, "Every patient gets a test and a prescription. Otherwise I get complaints."

I SOMETIMES GET emails from people who are uneasy about an article they've come across that contradicts my ideas, these two articles being good examples:

> www.huffingtonpost.ca/2016/01/28/schizophrenia-cause_n_9099128.html
> www.theglobeandmail.com/opinion/the-explosive-science-of-genetics/article28462603/

Because the articles imply that biology is or soon will be the key to understanding human behaviour, the articles are horribly wrong. To warm you up to their errors, I'll give you some preposterous advice. The next time you have dinner with a friend, rely exclusively on biological theories in deciding what you are going to say, and use the same biological approach to understand what your dinner partner says. Call on any brain nuclei, pathways, or neurotransmitters that you want. But you are forbidden to do what is usually done in social situations: no speculation about motives and no reliance on behavioural clues is allowed. It doesn't have to be dinner. Using the same biological tactic, you can try negotiating a business deal with a colleague, a prostitute, or the cashier in your supermarket. The fact is, you won't accomplish a thing, not even to arrange a meeting time.

There are plenty of examples of how using misplaced language can be daft: sending a thank-you card to a test tube in which a successful experiment has been done; assessing your boyfriend's genetic loading as a Valentine's Day tactic; giving absolution to an algebraic equation that has frustrated us. It's equally daft to attribute art to that part of our brain referred to as the reptilian hindbrain, or the glories of love to blind hormones, or madness to demonic chemicals.

Special circumstances call for special languages, so biological language works extremely well for biological matters; for arguing with your enemy it is useless. In the confessional we use a special language, that of sin, grace, absolution, repentance, penance, and forgiveness; in the genetics laboratory it's MZ and DZ twins, concordance, penetration, and loading; in a love nest it is poetry, beauty, miracles, and flowers. In the right circumstances, special languages work, if not perfectly, almost perfectly. The wannabe artists that make up only a small minority of psychiatrists also mix languages, but the languages they mix are all members of the social speculation family; they don't invoke or challenge biological issues. These psychiatrists bring to bear new angles on matters of social speculation. But even though modern psychiatrists often make the horrible error of using biological language for the social behaviour of the patients (as I said, try it out and you'll see that it's worthless), in the artistic and linguistically oriented psychiatrist's office, to compare good manners to hypocrisy may be worthwhile. (The psychiatrist might also try out the ideas that hypocrisy is a cunning strategy, is often a matter of human decency, is a revolutionary act, is boringly common, is a complex strategy for being sincere.)

The authors of the two articles I cited want to graft biology onto human behaviour, something that can't be done. A chemical in the brain is not in the same logical universe as telling a joke or remembering the flowers your wife carried on your wedding day. The people who wrote these articles are in certain ways smart—but not psychiatrically smart. There, they are idiots, and the only excuse I can make for them is that they are like *most* psychiatrists and neurophysiologists. They want to suggest that there is a competition between biology and psychology, the biologists possessed of the stupid idea that their side will win—even though they are as biologically inept in a social situation as anyone else who tries to rely on biology.

DR. KIFUJI IS part of a subculture that includes all those who think the stupid, confusing, and odd behaviours that all of us deal with sometimes and psychiatrists deal with often must be understood biologically even though their evidence cache is empty. Young psychiatrists aren't being taught that when there are no biological abnormalities, they should listen psychologically, see whether they can get a worthwhile conversation going. Members of the biology cult (without a doubt, the drug enthusiasts are a sub cult of psychiatry) haven't considered changing their way of thinking about patients, haven't realized that language changes everything. Its members have forgotten that in the absence of evidence, to say that a patient has a "disease" is correct only if they remember they are using a metaphor. If they insist they are referring to a tangible disease, they are voicing a wild opinion, not offering information based on evidence. To call this group of psychiatrists a subculture is the most accurate designation, but accuracy isn't everything; I also want to pin on them a label that includes disapproval. I therefore say that doctors like Dr. Kifuji who use dangerous drugs recklessly are members of a blood tribe, examples of herd behaviour and a pack mentality.

In chapter 5, I'll have more to say about subcultures, tribes, and pack mindsets, especially about our passion for adopting the styles of living we see around us, to live in harmony with the various subcultures of our world: married, sophisticated, atheist, sexpot, artist, revolutionary, expert-at-wrecking-one's-own-life, and so on, endlessly. But these are not just casual styles. Such identifications are fervent; hypnotized, we sleepwalk according to whatever fashions we've grabbed onto. Mark Twain summed this up nicely in 1901.

> I am persuaded that a coldly thought-out and *independent verdict* upon a fashion in clothes, or manners, or literature, or politics, or religion, or any other matter that is projected into the field of our notice and interest, is a most rare thing—if it has indeed ever existed.
>
> A new thing in costume appears—the flaring hoop skirt, for example—and the passers-by are shocked, and the irreverent laugh. Six months later everybody is reconciled; the fashion has established itself; it is admired, now, and no one laughs.[2]

The words that confirm membership in a cultural subgroup are innocent sounding: *fashion*, *style*, *taste*, *ritual*, *trend*, *way of life*. To these words I'll add another word, this time not innocent; in fact, it's insulting: *superstition*. To call a fashion a superstition doesn't require a leap

2 Mark Twain, "Corn-Pone Opinions," 1901 (First published posthumously in 1923; edited by Albert Bigelow Paine).

of the imagination; a fashion is superstitious because it is valued for no logical reason, valued because we are intensely social animals, inevitably drawn to living in ways similar or identical to people around us. To use the word *superstition* is to take a different angle on the more benign-sounding words I first used, an angle that matters because superstition blinds us, tempts us to join in on bad group thinking—racism, sexism, homophobia, cult indoctrination, and so on—very different from benign group enthusiasms such as cheering for our favourite team. Those who have signed on with a cultural subgroup do it because they either *believe in* or *feel obligated to behave* in the cultural style in question. This doesn't mean we necessarily like the actions we are caught up in. I hate it when I'm polite to a sycophant, a bully, or a fool, but since I'm caught up in the culture of politeness, I'm persuaded to behave politely. But I still like—and often prefer—other of my actions, parts of the culture that suit me, even if I follow them less often than actions I dislike in myself.

IT'S STRANGE THAT unless they tell me, I have no way of knowing the diagnostic habits of other psychiatrists; every psychiatrist uses diagnostic labels differently. Some think these labels point to real diseases; others, including me, are only dismayed by psychiatric labels. Patients give off hundreds of messages, a wealth of clues and more clues, and by offering a wealth of treatments and more treatments, we psychiatrists return the favour. In the rest of medicine, things aren't like that. There, clues point to material diseases, and all doctors can decipher these signs and symptoms: appendicitis, pneumonia, and prostatic hypertrophy usually aren't hard to figure out, and for each there are specific well-established treatments.

The psychiatrists who prepared the DSM-5 (*Diagnostic and Statistical Manual of the American Psychiatric Association*—a sacred text for psychiatrists in much of the world, the state-of-the-art diagnostic manifesto) admit that all psychiatric diagnoses are descriptive; none are to be identified with a cause. Yet almost all of my colleagues, especially those who work at the university, have not paid attention to this news. More serious than that, *they don't seem to have paid attention to their own patients*. The following quotation is from a book at the heart of psychiatric orthodoxy, a progress report on the DSM-5 planning process, which is an official publication of the American Psychiatric Association.

> ... the goal of validating these syndromes [i.e., psychiatric disorders] and discovering common etiologies has remained elusive ... not one laboratory marker has been found to be specific in identifying any of the DSM-defined syndromes. Epidemiologic and clinical studies have shown extremely high rates of co-morbidities among the disorders, undermining the hypothesis that the syndromes represent distinct etiologies. Furthermore, epidemiologic studies have shown a high degree of short-term diagnostic instability for many disorders. With regard to treatment, lack of treatment specificity is the rule rather than the exception.
>
> The efficacy of many psychotropic medications cuts across the DSM-defined categories. For example, the selective serotonin reuptake inhibitors (SSRIs) have been demonstrated to be efficacious in a wide variety of disorders, described in many different sections of DSM, including major depressive disorder ... twin studies have also contradicted the DSM assumption that separate syndromes have a different underlying genetic basis ...[3]

Were they even more honest, the writers would go beyond an admission; they would have shouted out these conclusions from the rooftops: *Hold your fire, colleagues. We don't have the evidence we thought would show up. We've stumbled and have relied on opinions rather than evidence. It's time to reboot, to rethink things, to go back to basics and use the scientific method to debunk a lot of what we've been saying.*

Confessions like this are buried—as is the above passage—among many pages of speculative jargon, hopes, and predictions, a tiny glimmer of honesty in a book whose authors also restate all the old orthodoxies and politically correct pieties. Since we need all the hope we can get, it's easy to miss such honest admissions. Undeterred by their own confessions and equally unfazed by years of futile effort—I

---

3 D.J. Kupfer, M.B. First, and D.A. Regier, eds., *A Research Agenda for DSM-5* (Washington: American Psychiatric Association, 2002), p. xviii-xix.

don't know nor do I ever expect to know of a single discovery—psychiatric scientists clamour for increased research funding. In homage to this madness, it says on the walls of the psychiatric hospital where I work: "Research Transforms Lives." The Menninger Clinic where I trained uses the same slogan.

The obvious conclusion is that if there is nothing to treat, there's nothing to say except to repeat that *there is nothing to treat*—although, as distinct from treatment, there's usually plenty to talk about. I find the above fragment of honesty from the *DSM-5* committee admirable, but those who wrote it have tarnished their honesty by going further, stating that these purely descriptive diagnoses are *reliable* and can be identified by many clinicians, a statement that implies they are real diseases. Not only are they wrong, they are ridiculous; any of us can, with a high degree of reliability, identify geniuses, fools, bankers, homebodies, Lotharios, derelicts, and athletes—categories that are also not diseases. What counts is *validity*, and without an objective marker, no valid disease can be pinned down. Just the same, biological psychiatrists are determined to find the cause, the etiology, of mad behaviour. These psychiatrists, often professors and researchers, ignore what they themselves know, that there are no objective data to study, no signs that would make a search for causes plausible. Psychiatrists are just plain peculiar, a tribe that is stubbornly ideological even though, because there are no objective things on which to do research, there is no way of applying the scientific method to their patients.

If, as the authors of the above quotation say, all treatments work for all psychiatric disorders, what in the world are we psychiatrists doing? Were it true that laxatives, insulin, cough medicine, antibiotics, and hydrocortisone cream all helped all medical patients, including those with diabetes, cancer, tuberculosis, and hyperthyroidism, all medical treatments would be suspect. But obviously they *don't work* for all medical conditions. Contrast this with psychiatry in which drugs, psychoanalysis, every form of psychotherapy, and electric shock *do work* in the treatment of every psychiatric disorder. And, I should add, acupuncture, herbs, astrology, homeopathy, chiropractic, eating seeds, grass, and nuts, yogic flying, and being reborn in Christ *also work* in the treatment of every psychiatric disorder—although a lot of psychiatrists haven't noticed. But Robert Burton noticed. In his classic book, *The*

Anatomy of Melancholy, published in 1621, Burton said, "1001 causes and 1001 cures." The repetitive cry, "It works!" makes it obvious that these are placebo cures. This reminder will offend some people, but it is undeniably true.

Here is more evidence of the dodgy status of psychiatric diagnoses, obvious once one thinks of it: traditional medical symptoms are referred to by saying the patient *has* something: pain, cough, fever, nausea; psychiatric symptoms are talked about by saying the patient *is* something: schizophrenic, nervous, depressed, obsessive; *has* versus *is*. If we say *is*, use the verb *to be*, we've decided that it is the *person* who is troubled, that no alien disease has seized hold of him. I, of course, go further. Rather than saying someone is schizophrenic, nervous, depressed, or obsessive, I've concluded that we'd be better off if we spoke adverbially, said that the person lives crazily (I'm so repulsed by the *schizo* word that, for the moment, I can't say it again), nervously, depressively, or obsessively, thereby emphasizing that he can be thought of as the agent of his own life. Obviously, the psychiatrist can't cure her patient of being who he *is*, but she might help him change his ways, using adverbs to describe his actions and beliefs. And that's what my patients say: "My doctor helped me to change." Still, this proves little—all events change us.

Many who visit a psychiatrist have decided in advance what they want—commonly psychotherapy or drugs. Few ask for ECT (electroconvulsive treatment), although I had one patient who loved it—just as he loved being humiliated by prostitutes. Since psychiatrists are doctors, it seems like nonsense to decide on a "treatment" before a diagnosis has been made, so we struggle—first, to invent well-defined diagnoses, and second, to establish criteria for applying specific treatments to the fastidiously designed diagnoses we've invented. But the fancy diagnoses are a lot of hooey. No demons have been discovered.

If there's no evidence of disease, the reasonable conclusion is that if we respect our patients' rights and if they ask for psychotherapy, we should agree; if they ask for pills, we should prescribe. After all, we don't criticize people who take the waters at Baden-Baden, seek out acupuncture, or have their colons irrigated; it's no one's business except the person seeking treatment. The right thing to do is tell the patient that although he may be suffering, there is no disease, but that there are drugs and talking treatments that can help; then, after a discussion, he can choose. But I wouldn't agree to do just anything asked of me; I'm a snob, scornful of primal therapy, meditation, behaviour therapies, or any version of the cure by love. I'm actually even more opinionated than that: I approve of only a narrow range of methods, and in my office I have nothing else on sale.

Since I'm steeped in the traditions of medical practice, treating identifiable diseases, I hate the fact that I have to struggle with this. This is democracy, relativism, and liberalism misunderstood and gone mad. To leave the choice of treatment to the patient robs me of my power; moreover, it robs my patient of his greatest comfort. My authority is what allows me to have a benign influence—a benign but magical influence—on my patients. To advocate authority is politically incorrect nowadays, but where else should a patient turn but to a socially designated authority figure? If your toilet won't flush, call a plumber; if you are getting divorced, call a lawyer.

Although the psychiatrist may relinquish her power to dictate which treatment is to be chosen, that doesn't mean that power is bad, although there is a climate of opinion on the loose that says power in its very nature is bad, something to be frowned upon. I don't believe it. If, for example, a woman is skilled at being feminine, isn't it splendid that she celebrates her power, a power that some seem to find vulgar, but which is obviously wonderful, thrilling, and superb? The same goes for sexy men, those to whom women flock—each holds a power that resembles charisma. The power of the doctor is less personal, a social attribution she uses for the benefit of her patient. It permits her to examine his nakedness, allows her to put instruments into his body, gives her the privilege of instructing her patient about therapeutic measures he ought to take, including drastic measures like surgery. This includes the power of the psychiatrist, whose words are to be taken seriously, often more seriously than would the same words uttered by friends or family.

Many placebos are harmless, including most over-the-counter remedies, the ministrations of massage therapists, naturopaths, and chiropractors (though I worry about spinal manipulation)—as long as they don't recommend against vaccination and other confirmed medical treatments. I have a report in front of me that says that 60 percent of medical doctors in the United States find giving placebos to be an ethical practice, despite professional rules that forbid this.[4]

Such rules are ridiculous. Doctors have always known that to do our work properly, some degree of medical magic is necessary, that the promise of help is why people visit us. Reassurance, for example, is an excellent medical practice, but its effectiveness is nothing more than a talking doctor's verbal magic. But I worry about some placebos, those given by charlatans who promise cures and charge high fees, not to speak of powerful drugs that have little efficacy, only dreadful side effects. Just the same, a medical ritual is called for, but what that ritual should be is up for grabs. I've opted for the talking-doctor ritual, the one that Socrates chose: "... to talk every day about virtue and the other things about which you hear me talking and examining myself and others, is the greatest good to man, and that the unexamined life is not worth living for a human being..."

Psychiatric oddness or unhappiness isn't like cancer and other medical disorders for which there are well-established treatments. Were a psychiatrist to treat her patient with acupuncture she'd be considered peculiar, but such an act wouldn't be dangerous neglect, as it would be were she to recommend that a cancer patient try acupuncture. Yet I hate the idea that a psychiatrist would recommend it. The reason it offends me is nothing more than my love of tradition: it's not the kind of thing we talking doctors do—or, more accurately, it's not the kind of thing we doctors have done until recently. If liberty demands that the psychiatrist should give her patient what he wants, yet if professional tradition says that she should not simply give her patient what he wants, what should the psychiatrist do?

AS DISTINCT FROM helping people with mental problems, I'll now attempt to describe how the treatment of real disease works. I'll start with an example of cancer cells, and with this example, I want to be

4 Will Dunham, "60% of MDs Find Placebos Ethical: Study," *Globe and Mail*, October 24, 2008, http://www.theglobeandmail.com/life/60-of-mds-find-placebos-ethical-study/article1350380/.

clear that I'm not being imaginative and subjective when I tell you that these cells have an objective existence. The fact is that in large masses these cells form tumours big enough to be seen with the naked eye; sliced, they can be studied under a microscope and touched, moved, and manipulated. Not only can the presence of malignant cells be objectively apprehended and diagnosed, the cells can be medically attacked through surgical, chemotherapeutic, and radiation procedures. They are honest-to-God tangible things. And with such diseases, the Aristotelian idea of objects (people) having qualities (diseases) works very well. Of course, cancer can also be attacked with prayer, meditation, and will power, but these methods aren't about objective facts; rather, they are about mind, beliefs, and spirituality.

Doctors diagnose, study, and treat many objectively real things. Infectious bacteria, glandular disorders, arthritic joints, and blocked coronary arteries are just a few examples. Treatments of such material ailments count as being effective only if they lead to material changes in the abnormal structures. For example, if after the day after his heart attack, a man announces he is better, no doctor believes this means the patient's diseased heart is cured. Medical improvement is not established by the patient's subjective opinion; it is determined by examining the heart, studying its electrical status, watching it function on an echocardiogram, and measuring the enzymes the damaged heart muscle leaches into the bloodstream. Yet when a depressed person tells his psychiatrist he is better (or checks a box on a questionnaire—questionnaires make opinion sound important), and if the psychiatrist is one of that breed who believes in psychiatric diseases, she assumes that the patient's report of improvement indicates a change in some disease process. Research on psychiatric treatments has nothing to go on except such questionable opinions. Because they are not based on evidence, opinions must always be tentative. If Tom Sawyer offers the opinion that warts are cured by stump water, few would take him seriously; if Alexander Fleming gives evidence—*objective* evidence—that penicillin cures staphylococcus infections, most would take him seriously. I remind you again that it comes down to *opinion* versus *evidence*.

After she's sized up the situation, the psychiatrist takes action. She delivers what's nowadays called treatment, although what the treatment should be is by no means clear. Psychiatry has given up on whips, straitjackets, bloodletting, and (mostly) electroconvulsive therapy. It's not that ECT does harm; running a marathon and a pummelling at the hands of a favourite dominatrix probably wipe out more neurons than a modern ECT machine. Harmless or not, apart from drugs, physical treatments are out of fashion. Besides, there's no scientific evidence of a "pathological" condition that can be altered by electric shocks. Yes, most of her patients will tell her they are better, but no good psychiatrist believes the rave reviews that so often come her way. (Charlton Heston once said to Laurence Olivier, "I've finally learned to ignore bad reviews." "Fine," Olivier replied, "now learn to ignore the good ones.")

I suspect the greatest hazard faced by psychiatrists is the disappointment when I remind them that they are being fooled by the dominatrix effect: all kinds of things make people feel better. Dominatrices are minor players in this game; commoner are cures through talking, pills, laxatives, and sea voyages. But it's hard to argue that these are real cures. The drugs that psychiatrists prescribe aren't nearly as effective as is commonly thought. It is well known, for example, that if effective at all, antidepressants are barely better than sugar pills.[5] As well, bias in the reporting of test results makes it impossible to know exact figures. And if we give these drugs to patients, might we be doing harm? If I shoot up, snort a line of cocaine, drink whiskey, or smoke pot, I'm creating abnormalities in my brain, although it's uncertain whether these changes are permanent. Psychiatric drugs also create brain abnormalities, and it is well known that some cause *permanent* abnormalities.[6]

---

5 See this thorough study: P.W. Andrews, J.A. Thomson Jr., A. Amstadter, and M.C. Neale, "*Primum Non Nocere*: An Evolutionary Analysis of Whether Antidepressants Do More Harm than Good." *Frontiers in Psychology* 3, no. 117 (April 2012), doi.org/10.3389/fpsyg.2012.00117.

6 See: Claudia Dreifus, "A Conversation with Nancy C. Andreasen: Using Imaging to Look at Changes in the Brain," *New York Times*, September 15, 2008, http://www.nytimes.com/2008/09/16/health/research/16conv.html?pagewanted=print.

5

Even the Gods Are Superstitious

Quisque suos patimur Manes
(We make our destinies by our choice of gods).
VIRGIL

I'VE ALWAYS MADE sure I have many kinds of patients—playwrights and paupers, divas and the despairing, maniacs, the mad, and the mundane. That's because these are the kinds of people who walk through our office doors; it's what most doctors' practices are like. Four groups of patients are as ordinary as all the rest. As I said before, only a few years ago the patients from these four groups were thought *not* to be ordinary; instead, it was believed that they were biologically abnormal, inferior to nice white males like me. These groups are blacks, Jews, gays, and women. Back then, the idea that they had bad genes seemed to be just as obviously true as it nowadays seems to be obviously wrong—genes that steered them down a life path not as dependable and valuable as mine. I'm appalled that my colleagues have to be reminded that when they say our patients' biology is abnormal, they are reacting to the culture of madness by extruding them in exactly the same way as were women, blacks, Jews, and gays a few decades ago—which is tantamount to creating a new variant on race, religion, or sex prejudice.

I now want to demote from centre stage a few things I like—for example, the plays of Shakespeare and the music of Beethoven. We're best off, I say, not arguing that these artists are "better" than modern artists. Lots of people don't like Shakespeare and Beethoven, preferring popular novels and the music of Bruce Springsteen. The only way I can argue that my literary and musical choices are better, that I am right and other people are wrong, is to set up a hierarchy: my taste is better than their taste. Like Plato, I'd have to argue that I am a philosopher king, that my judgment is worth more than someone else's. I say, don't set up aesthetic hierarchies. Stick with describing what's going on, that someone else's taste is *different* from mine. But don't discard hierarchical thinking; it's needed for moral issues, for dealing with evil people like rapists, killers, and thieves. I'm content to be arbitrary on that score and say that my moral code is better than their moral code, and I'm ready to argue the point. And I'm sure my moral code about how psychiatry ought to be practised is better than that of those who prescribe dangerous drugs and take away patients' civil rights. In the real world, it's often hard to choose between simply taking note of differences and taking note of right and wrong/health and sickness/better and worse. Should I have second thoughts about this? When it comes to plays, should I go back to insisting that those written by Shakespeare are better, while other plays are garbage? The answer is no.

We psychiatrists help individuals, but insofar as psychiatry is influential in our culture, we stand for something beyond the help we give when Mary, John, or Peter tell us their woes. The "something else" we stand for is a philosophy, one we psychiatrists don't publicize as much as we should—the philosophy that distinguishes radically between taste and moral judgment. None of us, ever, can evade making that distinction, that fundamental choice. Is this person's behaviour merely difference and uniqueness? Is this behaviour evil, something against which I must take a stand? And a much more iffy question: Is this behaviour sickness? In my conception of her, the psychiatrist is only a concentrated version of the wider world, caught forever between being reflective, thoughtful, and insightful, forever dithering and pondering things, and the opposite, being an agent of morality, force, will, and action.

If the assumption that psychiatric patients have biological abnormalities is wrong, we've got in our gunsights one of the great scourges of human life: prejudices like racism, sexism, and homophobia. When we think hard about this and study the wayward reasoning of psychiatrists who depersonalize and demean patients in this way, we learn something even more important. I'm not talking about merely behaving better—that would be boring, another superficial political correctness that would leave untouched the bad thinking that lies beneath our surface behaviour, thinking that could then be redirected against another group of citizens we decide to debase. I'm after the bad thinking that's in all of us, the almost automatic tendency to think that *I'm* okay and those who are religiously, racially, politically different—or in the case of psychiatric patients, socially different—aren't as good as I am. All forms of colonialism, slavery, racism, and most wars have depended on this line of thought. If we do this, we are like the Mayans of San Juan Chamula I'll describe in chapter 17, who find it acceptable to create a class of people who, once they've been defined as the enemy, become *los expulsados*.

Western society seems nowadays to be preoccupied by the idea that people should never be critical or cranky, should focus on kindness, empathy, and virtue. Under the premise that Africans are helpless and need to be bailed out—you understand, of course, that theirs is a "primitive" culture—many of these altruists preach the exportation of Western medical, moral, and cultural styles to Africa. They are blind to the obvious: if and when Western technology becomes a priority for them, African countries will see to it that they get it; if interested in Western cultural habits, they will adopt them. I'm not easily fooled, and I'm suspicious of virtuous moralizing. Humans, diseased as we are, are cunningly skilful at believing that virtue (for those in the West, that includes our obviously "better" technology and culture) is in us. We are equally cunning at believing that inferiority and wickedness are in others. Watching the evening news mocks claims of human virtue. Here are some killers, a list on which, no matter how difficult or painful, we must find . . . ourselves.

- Cromwell: six hundred thousand Irish (half the population of Ireland)
- Pol Pot: two million Cambodians
- Leopold II of Belgium: ten million Congolese
- Hutus in Rwanda: eight hundred thousand Tutsis

When people say, "Have a nice day," I want to respond with, "No thanks. I have other plans." But I keep quiet. If I tell people that years ago I gritted my teeth and drowned unwanted kittens, advocates of perfected kindness are shocked. Even setting traps for mice earns disapproving looks. But isn't kindness relative? If we were *all* kind, relative to whom would we appear kind? For example, would we be kind compared with immigrants, especially those who come from cultures with so-called Latin qualities and who are bad because they yell and throw dishes, behaviour supposedly typical of such "old-fashioned" cultures? Probably those with "Latin" cultural habits also give their children whacks on the bum, as I did fifty years ago; already then, my bum whacks were suspect. Are such cultural traits bad compared with our current ways, our hypocritical ways in which people apologize for political and legal reasons rather than because they're truly sorry for what they've done? Our ways in which we sit in front of computers drinking our morning orange juice and direct drones on killing missions?

The point is this: when we are certain we are on the road to goodness and virtue, we have in mind complementary groups of people who we are equally certain are evil or inferior, groups that we find it legitimate to oppress or, in the case of psychiatric patients, legitimate to "rescue" by suppressing them with drugs (against their will) or by locking them up (against their will). Guess what? Those we decide are evil or inferior always end up being people other than ourselves. Were it me in the dock, the one accused of yelling and throwing dishes, I'd mostly be exonerated, first because I have glib intellectual answers for those who want to judge me, and second, because I'm a nice, white citizen who talks exactly as do those tempted to judge me. Nor are British or Scandinavian immigrants judged. Even if we're not blatant in our racism, it's those other people who are judged, those with funny accents, from countries in collapse, or from some-place-or-other-*istan*, the ones who wear funny clothes and believe in funny deities. Claiming virtue = judging others.

It is true, of course, that we ought to be judged according to how we treat the weak, those who can't defend themselves—children, animals, the socially unhappy and troubled. When we try to behave, to give up our prejudices, it's easy to secretly continue our bad practices by concocting new categories of people we can scorn, substitutes for blacks, Jews, gays, women, and immigrants. The mad are easy to pick on, and if we devalue them, it's easier to think that we, the sane, are okay. Inferiority and bad genes, we can say, are in *them*. Since *they* are the aliens, our ways, our gender, and our race are okay. We psychiatrists are infected with pack behaviour, an infection against which the only vaccine is self-wrenching thoughtfulness. Psychiatry has always been a project in prejudice, which means that challenging the status quo isn't just an intellectual exercise. It's writing the stories of Martin Luther King, the Salem witch hunts, and Harvey Milk all over again. Because the mad don't speak up on their own behalf as articulately as blacks, women, and gays, changing the story will be hard to pull off.

Many argue that the medicalization of madness removes a widespread stigma. Yet I cannot imagine a worse stigma than being told that I am biologically or genetically abnormal, or that I have an abnormal brain. More stigmatizing still is to insinuate that, unlike you and me, crazy people aren't the authors or agents of their own lives; rather, they are victims of a disease/affliction and can't help what they do. The stigmatization won't end simply because we urge the world to stop thinking of the mad in these disgraceful terms, especially if we hypocritically urge tolerance, then tell patients they are abnormal. All too often we psychiatrists emphasize to the courts and the press that criminals suffer from mental disorders, underlining the common public idea that mental disorder equals wickedness. I'm not suggesting that informing people that madness is only another social practice will change anything; sadly, discrimination won't end no matter what we do or say. But if we psychiatrists, the God-experts, think about our own stigmatization of madness, we'll do better, especially if we speak to the public more honestly—especially if we God-experts speak to *ourselves* more honestly. Good thinking, talking, and writing influence the culture, and that's the aim. The things at stake are the symbols and symbolic statements we use to make sense of the world and of our own lives.

If—as Nietzsche teaches—instead of speculating about invisible diseases, complexes, and chemicals, we were to stick to description, to what is in front of our noses, we'd be further ahead.

> Oh, those Greeks! They knew how to live. What is required for that is to stop courageously at the surface, the fold, the skin, to adore the surface, to believe in forms, tones, words, in the whole Olympus of appearance. Those Greeks were superficial—out of profundity.[1]

My colleagues tell me that concern about social Darwinism is ridiculous, that even if it were true that psychiatric patients have a biological abnormality, this wouldn't cause trouble, lead anyone to think of them as inferior. They are preposterously wrong. I often hear that, on genetic grounds, parents discourage their child from marrying someone who, as they say, "is bipolar" or "has schizophrenia in the family." Where else but from doctors would they get the mistaken idea that these ways of life are biological, inherited, genetically based? The obvious conclusion is that psychiatrists should never, ever tell someone they have a genetic or chemical disorder—unless it's true. But were psychiatrists to comply with my demand, would this rob patients of a comforting story, one that gives relief because it says his troubles are not his fault, that it's a nasty biological flaw that he's been unlucky enough to inherit? Well, to start with, the story is a lie. Second, it's a story of hopelessness because if a disorder is genetic, little can be done. But if we talk differently, speak of how the patient has devised a worrisome narrative about what's going on, there's room for hope—it's possible to change one's mind; stories can be tinkered with. As I've noted, the comfort a person feels from the placebo effect is not to be sniffed at. While anything we doctors do is liable to induce the placebo effect, surely we can do better than telling a lie.

If I debunk my own powers, confess that there are no nasty brain chemicals and pathological psychological structures, confess that I'm a lapsed priest, have no pills, gestures, or magic phrases up my sleeve—none of it damages my ability to help. Why not? I can only speculate that my skepticism—and my bewilderment, amusement, uncertainty, curiosity—is part of a wider, infectious attitude that my patient becomes interested in, my unexpected style of conversation—interest in detail, metaphor, myth, grammar—a mindset that grabs his attention,

---

1 Friedrich Nietzsche, Preface for the second edition of *The Gay Science*, 1886.

a counterweight to the usual assumptions he lives by. It is notable that the placebo effect of inert pills occurs even if the doctor tells the patient that what she has prescribed are sugar pills. A common example of this occurs after I've had my car washed—as I drive off, the engine hums, and the car is sexier and more powerful. (Is this effect only on men?)

WHEN SOMETHING IS wrong, gurus tell us what's going on, give us the skinny on what ought to be done. Like gurus and other quacks, my psychiatric colleagues are confident: in the year 2016, no one admits what should be obvious to every psychiatrist: our patients suffer from "functional disorders." I hear no confessions that we don't know why our patients act as they do. Instead, in doctor's offices, online, on television, and in the newspapers, we are flooded with psychiatric opinion (propaganda, really, and since they believe what they say, it's propaganda *and* superstition), solemn tales of imaginary brain disorders and the cruel effect on patients of supposedly poisonous parents, spouses, and traumatic events. Because they are my colleagues and my pals, I'm embarrassed. It's idle chatter, of course, gossipy fun over cocktails or at dinner. Like everyone else, in social circumstances I enjoy targeting someone or something else, especially if it lets me off the hook. But as professional information, these opinions are hogwash. In truth, such psychiatric judgments are gross and moralistic, unworthy of a profession that has only one obligation: to help. I'm sorry to say this confirms that my colleagues are cultists.

The abnormal chemicals supposedly discovered by psychiatrists are nothing more than wild imaginings about the sources of the social practices of our patients, explanations so weak and so evidentially unsupported that no thinking person should be caught dead taking them seriously.

In contrast to biological/scientific psychiatrists, psychologically oriented psychiatrists work in the humanist tradition and rely on interpretation rather than pretending that they deal with demonstrable abnormalities. Talking doctors depend on the patient's cultural setting, behavioural analogies, verbal associations, the way the patient tells his history, evidence from other stories he has told and by quoting authorities—things of no interest to a scientist. Although these things constitute real evidence for why the patient lives as he does, they *prove* nothing; such interpretations are always open to revision and reinterpretation. But the biological-cult psychiatrists I'm complaining about have the bad habit of disqualifying the usual way of interpreting social behaviour, insisting on implausible truths about physiology, chemicals, and brain structures. Many talking doctors—literal-minded Freudians, Jungians, mindfulness practitioners, and others also have the bad habit of interpreting the world cultishly. All of them should know better.

Superstition is a nasty word, and I worry that by using it I'll lose your attention. Nevertheless, apart from reflexes, all our actions and thoughts are shaped by culture, and as such we blindly believe them to be right. In other words, they are cultural artifacts, styles, shortcuts for making the world functional. In order to disqualify what many of my colleagues say, I will call these artifacts what they are: culturally common superstitions. And with superstitions we must be careful; our actions may simply be enactments of cultural habits about which, upon reflection, we may change our minds. Since our actions are culturally embedded through and through, if we do change our minds and do something different, we will still have glommed onto a cultural practice—just a different one. Whoever claims to know scientific truths about psychiatry has deceived herself, is caught up in a superstition, has revealed that she is a citizen of Vanity Fair. In the view of many philosophers (the ones I agree with), science doesn't tell us the truth; scientific theories are never "true." They are theories only—fallible, usually well tested and fairly reliable but ready to be replaced at any time by theories that work better, theories that will also be replaced when an even better theory comes along. This alternative claim about science isn't brand new or a real truth about science; it's just something plenty of philosophers assert is a better way of thinking about science. Rather than the correct idea, it's another culturally known idea, albeit not as well known as thinking that science equals truth.

Superstition is far more widespread than we imagine, and the superstitions of psychiatrists resemble superstitions held by all of us. When the superstition stigmatizes people by suggesting that those who act in a weird or unhappy way have abnormal brains, and when this leads doctors to prescribe drugs that damage their patients' brains (I won't get into things like beheading people, tearing out their hearts on the altars of Mexican pyramids, and dropping napalm bombs), I intend the word *superstition* to wound those who think this way, sting them in the hope they may change their minds. These distinctions are not as finicky as you may think; in fact, they are quite obvious. Since they can never be tested, no non-scientific psychiatric theories could ever be relied on. Scientific theories welcome being debunked and their replacement by better theories. In other words, they aren't the truth either.

I'm hard on psychiatrists in other ways. I insist that, differing from what goes on in day-to-day life, our main tactic should *not* be to use supportive and reassuring methods. In regular life, things like support and reassurance are important; thank goodness that people tell us to have a nice day, assure us when there's trouble at work that our boss is an ass, suggest that when we've got the blues our hormones are out of whack. "You need to get more exercise," people say when our woes get us down. "Let's have a drink some night" or "Get rid of that jerk. He'll always screw you around that way." Many of us think Ouija boards and astrology are nonsense, yet if they are harmless and comfort someone, why judge them harshly? Dietary advice, fitness trainers, a massage, a new outfit, teeth whiteners, vitamins, and a tonic all make us feel better. Art and music, clubs and sports, public lectures and travel—all keep us going. And we need to be kept going because life is not a picnic. A psychiatrist gets called on only when the crucial support systems of everyday life don't work, so it would be stupid if the psychiatrist did the same things as everyone else: give advice and platitudes; offer placebos or another bromide.

Except in emergencies, the psychiatrist isn't in favour of pep talks—or she shouldn't be. Instead, she encourages her patients very differently—the difference is in her attitude. The psychiatrist's every action should demonstrate vigilance; whether her patient is palsy-walsy, lackadaisical, lazy, or a determined pessimist, she must take seriously everything he says and does. And she doesn't give up. She is determined to discuss, study, analyze, and clear up everything that's said, every facial expression and gesture, every tone of voice she's able to spot. She does give advice, but it's not ordinary advice, not explicit. Instead, her manner and her attitude do the speaking, suggesting, "Take yourself seriously. Your every breath, your every twitch, is worth attending to."

EVERYTHING WE DO is a story told or enacted. If Einstein invents the theory of relativity, it's a story, a scientific narrative; if you propose going on vacation, it's a narrative; if you argue with me, we are throwing competing narratives at each other (or else it's a narrative about how people can throw competing narratives at each other). If you argue that the basic stuff of life is material substance, that life is nothing but an idea in the mind of God, or that there is nothing we can be aware of except narratives—those are all narratives. There's no arguing with people who hold to their beliefs absolutely because such convictions, to them, are self-evident truths—their god, their religion, their prejudices, or their superstitions—that are fixed firmly in their minds. And invariably we latch onto the narrative that represents a cultural subgroup we've decided is the right one for us, whose way of thinking about things suits us. I've already pointed out that the phrase *cultural subgroup* is sometimes too benign, that the term also refers to cults, tribes, fashions, superstitions, group hysteria, and wolf-pack behaviour.

These are complicated words, especially the word *superstition*. Most of us in the West think our culture is modern and not superstitious, especially compared with Africans, Asians, and other non-Europeans; we are sure that, if we *are* superstitious, it's to a far lesser degree than it was once upon a time. Of course, Asians and Africans also talk this way about us. When they buy a house, Cantonese Chinese in Toronto have what I consider weird and complicated geographic demands regarding its north-south-east-west orientation; they, in turn, think *I* am weird, that I am a *gweilo* (ghost, foreign devil), and they think of me as less human than they are. We don't say *gweilo* but prefer to use the words *primitive* or *underdeveloped* or *third world*. Tellingly, we insist that superstition is a characteristic of other cultures, not ours, that we live in the "developed/non-superstitious" world.

Do we really want to fall back on the idea that some cultures are primitive whereas ours is advanced? That women, Africans, Jews, Muslims, and other foreigners are savages, while the rest of us are sophisticated? That a tribal culture isn't as valuable as an urban culture? The truth is that taking care of your ancestors' bones is very practical to certain Asians and Africans. Similarly, talking on a cell phone is very practical to a large part of the rest of the world. Building grand hospitals is practical, isn't it? And in some cultures making an appointment for the fetish-man to come to the house ten days from now is undoubtedly practical. Because everyone tells their secrets to the fetish-man, the money that disappeared will have been returned by the time he arrives.

If you are interested in health food, tasting menus, fitness clubs, annual physical examinations, the *New York Times*, vitamins, supplements, chiropractors, psychiatrists, Dr. Phil, the latest fashion, a successful career, knowing Greek myths and Nietzsche, then you are superstitious. It doesn't matter whether you fudge by calling these things interests or hobbies, whether you attribute high importance to them, attribute no importance to them at all, whether you denigrate them or find them boring—it's all based on superstition. How do I know? Because my infallible god, the one upon whom my own superstitious opinions depend, tells me that all of your social acts are, to you, sacred, precious, religious, and superstitious. If they weren't, you wouldn't undertake them. All actions depend on a decision and a belief that a particular choice is correct; whatever you do, you've decided it's right. Although sometimes you are flexible, ready to change your mind, and open to other opinions, at other times you're rigid, certain that the way you've done something is the only right and proper way to do it.

Superstition, style, and ritual are different things, but all are rooted in adherence to a social tradition, a commonality with one or another form of tribal behaviour. To me, my professional *style* is the right way to behave in my office. That style is to be strictly business, always be cautiously informal and ironic, make interpretive meta-comments when I have a chance—that's what I'm paid to do—boldly enough that patients are sometimes taken aback, at other times impressed.

My style is also a *ritual*, a routine and precious way of doing things, something I've sanctified not because I believe in it absolutely but because... because... well, okay, I *do* believe in it absolutely. Making my methods sacred keeps me imagining my work is precious and fine. But in fact, mostly what it does is keep me a bit safer from slipping up in the way I apply my methods. It also fulfills a fantasy of mine: I'm godlike in the way I do my work. (I call this a fantasy so you won't jump on me; deep down, it's worse: I really believe it.) Fundamentally, superstition is a belief that is irrational; despite my complaints that psychiatrists have superstitious beliefs about madness and craziness, my beliefs about how I practise indicate that I am as superstitious as the next guy.

If style, ritual, and superstition—and fashion, tradition, and so on—are at root the same thing, we come to a destabilizing and hilarious awareness: every social practice is the enactment of a superstition. Flinching when someone strikes out at you is an innate reflex; swearing at a tough guy is a social practice based on the superstitious idea that swearing at a tough guy is the right thing to do. If Janie Canuck's style is to swear at people, the way she does it is ritualized, and she superstitiously believes it to be the best way to behave when annoyed. The evangelical materialist is also holding to a superstition, so messed up in her thinking that she wants to explain Mona Lisa's smile by studying the paint used by Leonardo in his portrait of her. Christopher Hitchens's rants against religion are also evangelical, and although aware of his own imperfect humanity, he doesn't figure out that what he is getting worked up about is an institution that is, like his set of practices, only an example of the commonplace. My idea that every idea is up for grabs is itself a superstition, as is my *conviction* that I can change a particular human habit that will never and can never go away. We can use gentler words, call these *opinions*, but if the materialist Hitchens and I are convinced of our point of view, we're selling something stronger than an opinion: superstition, religion, an absolutism. We believe in our superstitions because our god has revealed the truth to us.

As opposed to opinion, convictions are dangerous. Convictions that women have it coming to them, that children should not be deprived of sex, and that psychiatric patients have diseases, lead to rape, to pedophilia, and to dangerous drugs being given to crazy people. I suggest that both the materialistic Christopher Hitchens's ghost and I should surrender up our convictions and switch to saying that these are some of the opinions that are popular today. But I wouldn't say that about murder or rape. Those, I denounce. When it's only today's opinion, we can say that materialism is a good foundation for certain kinds of thinking, something for those who want to try it out, want to see whether there's a payoff. When we come upon strong beliefs, we're best off being skeptical. Such attitudes, if transformed from convictions to cautious opinions, allow us to change our minds. Watch out for fanatics, I say, especially the fanatics that go by your name and mine.

A last word: Have you caught me out yet? When I suggest opinion in place of conviction, have you noticed I am imposing my fanaticism on you, the fanaticism that says that everything is to be doubted, that everything should be looked at as mortal opinion? Even though you've caught me out, I stand by that opinion and that particular taste because I believe it has a payoff. There's no psychiatric payoff to materialism, nor is there a social payoff to denouncing religion (even if the religion is a sacred belief in medical progress and perpetual health), but if we're careful, and if we realize that thinking is fallible, there is a payoff: we will be less vehement in our stigmatization of the mentally troubled—the crazy, tragic, and weird people who come to the attention of psychiatrists.

6

The Total Institution

The nail that sticks out gets hammered down.
JAPANESE SAYING

TOTAL INSTITUTIONS are conceived idealistically, and in many respects, their care for disabled people is more than competent—it's terrific. My brother Ernie, disabled by a stroke at age thirty-five—he's now seventy-eight—lives in a nursing home in which the residents are fed, bathed, and tidied up much more conscientiously than I had expected. Even though many patients are incontinent, rarely are there horrible smells. Ernie lives in an obviously archetypal world, and to him a total institution or heaven on earth look much alike. It's not that he sees nothing but bare-naked archetypes; it's that his world is simplified: most of his stories are told by using a single word. For example, when he first met Jill, my daughter-in-law, he sat beside her on my couch and explained to her who the family members in my living room were.

Ernie pointed at the first person. "Pretty good, pretty good," he said.

Then, in a booming voice, he identified the next person: "Divorced, divorced."

The person farther along: "Alco-holic, alco-holic."

Next over: "Fifty-fifty."

And the next: "Perfect."

Before being institutionalized, Ernie lived in an apartment, where every Sunday morning I brought his groceries. Speaking loudly on the elevator, he sometimes embarrassed me by saying things we're not supposed to say:

"Nigger, nigger." (He had watched the basketball game the previous night.)

"The boss, the boss." (He had seen President Obama on TV the previous night.)

"Millionaire, millionaire." (This usually meant Lady Gaga or another popular performer that he'd seen on TV.)

"Finished, finished." (Someone was dying; an athlete was past his prime; a marriage was in jeopardy.)

As you will have noted, Ernie perseverates—the medical term for uttering the same word repeatedly—perhaps a way of consolidating archetypal images and ideas. When he still lived in his own apartment, here's how he did it one Sunday morning before I did his shopping. As always, I phoned in advance and asked what he needed. Although he couldn't name many items, he gave me cues that, because I'm familiar with his limited speech, I was usually able to figure out.

"White, white," he said one day.

"Do you need eggs, Ernie?" I said.

"No, no!" he said. "You know—white, white!"

"Milk? Do you need milk?"

"Trouble, trouble. You know, you know."

"Mayonnaise, Ernie? Do you need mayonnaise?"

"You know. You know. *When I shit!*"

"Oh," I answered. "You need toilet paper."

"Right," said Ernie, with relief in his voice. "Mayonnaise."

In one respect, total institutions don't do well: disruptive social behaviour, even if only a nuisance, isn't tolerated. When residents or inmates are irritating or are pests, as Ernie can be, the staff of nursing homes, jails, group homes, and psychiatric hospitals believe, like Dr. Kifuji, that they must "do something," and for this they need the help of a doctor, on whom they rely thoughtlessly and cunningly. The problem of exuberant or unpredictable behaviour is passed on to a doctor, someone who can both make decisions about the problem and quell the unattractive behaviour because she can redefine it as disease. We're all inclined to do this. For example, if your child has a behaviour problem, you might ask a doctor about it. And if she says to give the child a pill, you may well follow her instructions. And the side benefit is that you're off the hook, and responsibility is on the doctor's shoulders. In a total institution, what happens next is that, because of the headaches residents create for the staff, the doctor prescribes powerfully sedating drugs for the problem resident (shouldn't she, instead, prescribe Tylenol for the staff?). Pesky behaviour is not a medical issue in any moral or scientific sense; rather, it is that the doctor is frustrated because she doesn't know exactly how to respond to the team of helpers who have presented the problem to her. All too often, the final response is a drug that subjugates a pesky patient, chemical control instead of struggling with a problem that, more often than not, is nothing more than a nuisance.

Even though in a wheelchair and despite limited speech and intellect, Ernie is outgoing, cheerful, and energetic. When I visit, he tells me the news, mostly single words that identify the status of various staff members—married, divorced, has or doesn't have children, nurse, aide, cleaner, interested in sports, boss. Although most other residents of the nursing home are quiet or silent—only a few wail unhappily—Ernie's intensely outgoing manner makes him different. Because he is entertainingly social, staff members like him. But Ernie is also a problem: he demands that people be involved with him; he takes up the staff's time, distracts them from their tasks, and speaks in a loud voice.

How are these so-called problems solved? Since the nursing home has a doctor, Ernie's behaviour is reconceived; instead of saying that Ernie is a pest and an irritation, they say he is sick and needs treatment. The nursing home doctor plays her part and prescribes a pill. The pill is nasty, one of the antipsychotic drugs that subdues people, slowly but surely destroys neurons, and incrementally produces metabolic syndrome, a form of widespread physiological dysfunction that affects all who take them. Indeed, the pills have made Ernie fat and quiet, and in despair I think, "Oh, my God, they've pithed my brother. What should I do?" As medical students, we pithed frogs by inserting a needle into the base of their skull, thereby severing their spinal cord. This blinded the frogs and wiped out pain sensation. We students could then experiment on the frogs' various reflexes. The frogs, like the patients in nursing homes and psychiatric hospitals who have been "pithed" with powerful drugs, were easy to manage, and as we told ourselves, had been managed humanely.

The staff had other tricks. Previously, Ernie walked with a cane, but within weeks of arriving at the nursing home, he no longer had a cane but was in a wheelchair. Could this have been a fiendish and diabolical strategy to make Ernie more helpless than he already was? Because he was given huge, calorie-rich meals and was no longer active, Ernie quickly became fat. Did they want him fat so he would be even less mobile than the wheelchair made him, therefore easier to manage? It would have been a cinch to restrict Ernie's diet so he didn't become obese, but despite my reminders, nothing changed.

In nursing homes and in other total institutions, full citizenship of the patient is rejected, inequality taken for granted. I hate the drugs given to annoying people like Ernie, especially their dreadful side effects. But the drugs are not the core problem; rather, it's human folly—the determination to wipe out unconventional or disruptive behaviour (almost inevitable in total institutions) by making it into a medical problem, then suppressing the behaviour with a pill—not to speak of wheelchairs and unhealthy diets. Like most people, I hate it when people breach my tranquility, but most of the time the problem is not the person who has disrupted me but my own impatience.

I've talked to the staff about Ernie's medications and they ruefully explained that Ernie had poor impulse control, saying what I've heard from ward staff dozens if not hundreds of times when, on inpatient units of psychiatric hospitals, I too pithed people by prescribing antipsychotic drugs. Every morning after the ward staff meeting, I wrote prescriptions, vaguely aware that something was fishy about subduing patients, that I was a puppet acting out my role in a psychiatric culture—a thoughtless, therefore wicked psychiatric culture in which subdued patients are the ideal, a bit like the anatomy lab where quiet, subdued cadavers are the ideal. This pithing function is the major assignment given to psychiatrists and other doctors who work in group homes, nursing homes, hospitals, and jails. I feel strongly that doctors should *refuse* to do this, be *shamed* into no longer doing this, be *forbidden* to do this.

The same subjugation is routinely applied to psychiatric patients, and were the curse of psychiatric diagnosis wiped out, it would be easier to stop the subjugation. Because they are extreme, the mad affect us powerfully, which makes it hard to think clearly about their actions; they sidetrack us, and instead of letting them find their own way, we patronize them, quiet them down. When we talk to insane people, we retreat from ordinary interactions, baffled and blocked from doing what we usually do in social situations. And doctors have another reaction, a medical one—a determination to treat the cause of such behaviour, even though the cause being treated is purely imaginary.

Ernie hates the effect the drugs have on him, but he can't argue his case. I could make a fuss, but nowadays I rarely mention my concerns to the staff; my cowardice means that someone else will one day have to take on this battle.

7

The Hospital

... attention by a good nurse may be just as important as a major operation by a surgeon.

DAG HAMMARSKJÖLD, Swedish diplomat, second secretary-general of the United Nations

MARCH 16, 2014

Dear Dr. Warme[1]

I have been seriously harmed by psychiatrists. I will tell u my story and see if u can help me... In 1995 I was taking care of my children, abused by my common law, conjured up the fact that he was a pedophile, and that my Mom was a pedophile as well. I went to the woman's shelter and they called the police and took me into the psych ward at the L— regional Hospital. I was, at that point, calling the L— Police reporting my suspicions that my common law might have killed two people that were missing. To this day I still believe that he did something to my older daughter but that he did not kill anyone.

They placed my children in a foster home and told me that I had to take the meds in order to get my children back. I remember that the medication did not help me and actually harmed by brain. I was so tired and gained a lot of weight. I could no longer look after

1 Ms. Chan's letter has been transcribed verbatim, including errors. Name of hospital, city, and journal and other details are withheld.

my children and sent them to daycare for others to look after them. When I stayed in the hospital they said that medication was not good in breast milk and I thus stopped breast feeding. I have a University education and know stuff. I know that that screws up bonding.

I have went through a lot of hardship since then and have figured lots out. I am 43 years old and have recently moved back to R— where my children live with there Father. I have lived there for 6 months and have really gone down hill. I have wrote 2 suicide letters so far and know of a way to kill myself. My children dont come and see me and visit me. I cannot work. I have gotten something done to my face, a laser, and in my opinion it harmed my face... I have found out for myself that people with schizophrenia should not get it done because it is too shocking and because of the meds... As you can tell from my writings how disjointed my thoughts are.

I tried street drugs and found out that those on meds should not do drugs. I have extensive brain damage from that and from going on and off of meds to get a high dopamine because that is what I knew of and have done damage to my knees.

In my opinion if someone would have spoke to me in 1995 about my suspicions and let me have a rest and interfered with their Father and his behaviour I would never be in my condition with a messed up head, a messed up face and a messed up body. When I was on meds I gained so much weight I have a mid-section that hangs down.

I went off of my meds after 11 years, suffered brain damage from doing so and then moved. My dopamine was so high I began to believe in the pedophilic stuff again. I lost my children and was very very delusional. Began to believe hollywood was watching me and the local radio station. That they were making license plates for me and that people were telling me what to do by the traffic. I would never have become this way to a point where my dopamine was so high if my dopamine wasnt reduced to such a point for over 11 years...

I know the Charter of rights and freedoms. I have the right to freedom of thought, dignity, choice and most of important a family. I have no family to take care of but to give money to and to drive to. When I was quizzing my younger daughter of possiby being sexually abused by her Father they put out a court order for me that I was to not have contact with them and prevented me from seeing the school and to go to there place for 1 year...

Now there is zero bondage with me and my children. I just observe them, I have zero desire to be with them. I can not work and think about my face all of the time. I cannot get my children to be with me because I am not stabilized on my meds and that is in disrimination of those who are mentally ill to have a family.

I have just seen someone from the Schizophrenia Centre and she said those that have schizophrenia lose there brain power but in my opinion it is from the meds. My choice has been taken from me, my dignity, my thought, my opinion and my family was denied from me. From the side effects I experienced from the meds it impeded with my dignity. This is Canada and I am a person and was a person and deserved to be treated with dignity. Antipsychotics take that away...

Talking to someone reduces their dopamine and that is treating them with respect and dignity. Not giving them meds and ignoring what they have to say. Giving them meds reduces their stay in the hospital and makes their care quick. If I kill myself you will here of me in the news so please release this information of what I know so that my children will know what was done to me. I was born in a time of psychiatrists and their meds and have had my life ruined because of it. Medication and human beings don't mix...

I would like to whole system to be exposed and I would like psychiatrists to wake up to what they do to their patients. I was a fly on the wall in 1995 and people squashed me with their fly swatter of meds.

I was a [her profession], I was a research assistant and did not become this way because of schizophrenia. I am published in the Canadian Journal of L— if you want to look me up. Thank you for reading this. I dont care if your brain shrinks. Maybe I am the devil and want to destroy this way of psychiatrists and will be a devil if it works but what am I to do. Kill myself. Meds were not the answer to me and from what Ive told you my freedoms were violated. I would like to be a study object and for people to learn from me. I am currently on meds but my brain is destroyed. I cannot read, listen to most music, or exercise to my full strength...

Sincerely,
Wilma Chan

Unsurprisingly, Ms. Chan is in a total institution, a psychiatric hospital, and her description of her plight is all too accurate. Doctors and nurses who work in hospitals acclimatize, soon learning to cope with blood and guts, wounds, excrement, exudates—and even with death. But they do not acclimatize to the strange behaviour of psychiatric patients. And because of that, the story of Wilma Chan breaks my heart. It is the story of a life gone bizarre, savaged, lost, and worst of all, a life that is still aware—aware that she is an outcast to whom people react with revulsion. Wilma Chan and those of her tribe are universally treated as lesser citizens. And if reading her email makes anyone think that she is truly a lesser citizen—not blatantly, but through our actions—one who should be issued more pills and told she has a disease called schizophrenia, I'm hoping you will rethink what you're up to and where your ideas come from.

Ms. Chan's email arrived today; she wrote because she had read one of my books. I have no idea who she is. But to anyone who has worked in a psychiatric hospital, her tale is all too familiar. Later the same day, she left me a voicemail, something about her willingness to be a research subject if I or some researcher would take her on. The phone number was from a city thousands of kilometres from where I live and work in Toronto. Such a letter reminded me of another important lesson the psychiatrist has to learn: paying attention to how we, ourselves, react to our patients, our most difficult duty. Self-examination, if we can do it at all, is arduous, endless, and inevitably incomplete.

For example, my first reaction was to imagine Ms. Chan as a derelict lookalike, unclean, wearing a shapeless dress that did nothing to hide obesity, droopy boobs, and hairy legs—at least that's what I first thought I thought. But secretly, I had another thought, the same thought I'll attribute to Ralph Greenson in chapter 11 when I describe how he approached his work with Marilyn Monroe: *Maybe Ms. Chan is an Asian siren, one of those innocent-eyed, sweet, pure girls with golden skin and delicate underwear—waiting for Prince Charming (me) to awaken her.* Yes, like many of us, I'm powerfully influenced by my fantasies, and I was hoping upon hope that Wilma Chan was a lonely Bangkok bargirl in disguise, waiting to be saved. What psychiatrists say out loud is different: "She is sick and needs to be on an antipsychotic drug." Yes, the "she has a disease" stuff has the same hurricane power and is as romantic and potent a fantasy as the sex and rescue stuff.

March 16, 2014

Dear Ms. Chan,

I've picked up your phone message. As you can imagine, it's unlikely that we could ever work together. The distance is too great. But let me say a couple of things.

First, I have a question for you to think about, not because the question has an answer, but because it might get you thinking, learn a few things about yourself. It's the kind of question all of us ought to keep in mind if we're looking to change our lives. Here it is: "How did you get people to put you in hospital?" I urge you to think about this every day of your life because it's the most important question of all.

What other people did and why they did it is beside the point. Except for the things we do to influence them, neither you nor I can do anything about what others think or do. Thinking about *my* nuttiness is about the only hope I've got for changing my life, and thinking about *your* nuttiness is the only hope you've got for changing yours.

As far as your damaged face and brain are concerned, I have no comment. If they are damaged, there's nothing to be done and you'd be best off concentrating on something that *could* make a difference, namely, the question I mentioned above, the question of how you got people to lock you up, give you pills, restrict your life, etc. Their personal reasons are irrelevant because, my friend, it's mostly in your hands.

Good luck to you.

GW

I think my email hit the right tone. Even though supportive and polite, you can see that I pushed her, urged her to notice things in her story that so far she had been ignoring. Although I was acting as her guru, shaman, and talking psychiatrist, I was also acting as a theatre critic, suggesting a rewrite of a script that wasn't working.

ONE FLEW OVER THE CUCKOO'S NEST was the first film ever to win all five major Academy Awards, including Best Picture. Yet it's not a portrayal of life on a real psychiatric ward either then or now. It's a myth and a fairy tale, a caricature of psychiatry, our dirty linen, the linen that psychiatrists want to think is immaculate. The film blew psychiatry's cover—the first time I saw it I hated its insulting portrayal of psychiatry—and exposed psychiatry's moralistic reaction to psychiatric patients, clumsily masked by surface civility and professionalism.

By suggesting that the overt actions of Nurse Ratched (Rat-shit?) and Randle McMurphy—the Louise Fletcher and Jack Nicholson characters—represent what really happens on psychiatric wards, the film can mislead. Such obvious mistreatment hasn't happened in the West for many years and wasn't happening when the film was made. The real horror is not raw, not blatant, not obvious, as depicted in the film. In reality, the calm civility found on psychiatric wards is insidious, hiding what's actually going on. Although the employees and the inmates in the film's hospital are *not* civil and the war between Nurse Ratched and the patients is easy to see, on real psychiatric wards these poisons are hidden, lurking behind surface courtesies and the wrong type of professionalism—the wrong metaphor. Those of us who work on such wards try hard, yet we offend against what doctors and nurses ought really to do.

Here's my imagined scenario of what happened to Wilma Chan in the months or years before she wrote her letter. Immediately, she would have been addressed by her first name, an uncalled-for intimacy. To my chagrin, even old people in hospitals are denied their titles, their honorific Mr., Mrs., or Ms. On the other hand, even if thirty years younger than their patients, doctors are honoured with their full title. Most psychiatric patients are wretched and need plenty of validation, which is why addressing an older patient as Agnes or Fred appalls me—although it doesn't seem to appall anyone else. And it's not just older patients; it is professionally important to address *all* patients by their titles; the immediate use of first names is akin to calling someone *tu* in France or *du* in Germany when first meeting them. My revulsion with this impertinence is clear from how I've practised; I've never called an adult patient by his or her first name. *Cuckoo's Nest* follows this practice. In the film, Nurse Ratched addresses all patients by their titles, as was customary in those days. But her manner, tone, and style all give her away—her purpose is mockery and bossiness.

I remember those dictatorial head nurses. I don't know whether they still exist, but my evil mind suspects they have won the battle and we submissive psychiatrists have fallen in line, agreeing to control all behaviour on psychiatric wards that is a nuisance, is unusual, or hurts someone's feelings—almost exclusively with drugs.

WILMA CHAN WOULD have been admitted against her will. She probably talked about herself freely, perhaps obsessively, blurting out her crazy ideas that her husband and mother were pedophiles, that her husband might have killed two people, and that she had told this crazy stuff to her children. To those who believe in schizophrenia, she would be said to have obvious signs of the disease, delusions about her husband and mother, suspiciousness, and poor judgment about what should be told to children. Her hospital doctor would have interviewed her, made a diagnosis, and prescribed antipsychotic medication. Even before Ms. Chan was examined, this series of events could have been predicted—antipsychotic drugs are automatically prescribed for people like her, although it would never occur to Ms. Chan's doctor that what she, the doctor, was doing was *pre*scripted. Within a few days, Ms. Chan would have become quieter, definitely subdued. As is often true, she probably looked disconnected, spooky, or zombie-like, in a sleep-walking-yet-awake state, the common side effect of antipsychotic drugs.

Even if the hospital were modern, Wilma Chan would be spending most of her time sitting on the ward, often watching television. She almost certainly would talk to other patients, may have befriended one or two, but mostly she would be doing nothing, weakened and tired because of the drugs she was given. To be friendly and comforting, some of the staff would have talked to her, but this would occupy a tiny part of the day. Once or twice a week, there might be group therapy, and a social worker might come by. There is little to do on such wards: no shopping, no housework, no employment, no children to care for, no bills to pay, no errands, no appointments, no car to drive. *And no responsibility, the thing that motivates us, impels us to live.*

Recently, I hurt the feelings of a clergywoman when I said I didn't think chaplains were necessary in psychiatric hospitals. "I'm a chaplain at a hospital," she told me. "It's important that the patients' spiritual needs be attended to." My response: "Of course. So, like other people, they should go to church if they want their spiritual needs attended to." This lack of responsibility guarantees that psychiatric wards are socially poisonous—frustrating, depressing, frightening—in plain English, demoralizing hellholes. Other medical wards demand that patients take responsibility, sit up the day of abdominal surgery, wiggle fingers and toes. Because I'm physically fit, I was sent home to take care of myself three days after having both my knees replaced; the staff even made me walk on the day of my surgery. It wasn't fun, but the message was clear: you are not an invalid. Walk, and take care of yourself.

When I was a medical student, patients in mental hospitals—they were called asylums—had to work. They did laundry, grew their own vegetables, milked the cows, and scrubbed and polished the floors (they should have been paid for their work, of course, but they were not). Somehow, in the intervening years, it was decided that such duties infringed on their rights, and today, psychiatric patients are allowed to do few of the things that would give them self-respect. We forget that responsibility is an aspect of liberty, the freedom to manage one's own life or, better, the freedom that springs from being treated as competent. Liberty isn't just fun, of course; it includes effort, duty, and thinking things over, but the payoff is a sense of worth. Unfortunately, liberty has become a word that, nowadays, sounds like a slogan or a cliché—unfortunate because it is the best word for what the psychiatrist aims to give her patient. It's not licence, but the awareness that, apart from a short list of socially intolerable behaviour, her aim is to let her patient become who he himself wants to be.

A medical degree isn't needed to understand the desocializing effects of institutions. Even though it's a long-established custom to think of patients as damaged, it's inexcusable. It's also grotesquely naïve. The idea that Ms. Chan is damaged comes from *her*. *She* is the one who says her brain is damaged; *she* is the one who says she is a passive victim of wicked family members; *she* is the one who claims to be controlled by Hollywood, radio messages, and traffic. Because Ms. Chan thinks responsibility for her thoughts and actions is located in others doesn't mean we should believe her. "You have to walk, today," we should tell her, "wiggle your toes, sit up, think about how you attribute your troubles to other people, to things wrong with your brain, and to the radio." Instead, the common practice is to agree with her—"It's your brain"—and silence her with suppressive drugs.

Ms. Chan wouldn't have known what would happen in the hospital. She probably complained that the hospital had no right to hold her and that the drugs were damaging her brain. It would have been reported at the morning staff meeting that her delusions were persisting, that she had developed the delusion that the drugs were damaging her. Well, the truth is that the drugs *do* damage the brain, and all doctors know this—it's basic knowledge. But the tradition that leads doctors to instinctively prescribe antipsychotic drugs immunizes them against worrying about side effects. It's the way things are done. "Side effects are a risk with every treatment," their thinking goes.

The sociology of the ward depends on the idea that patients are sick. Therefore, whatever patients do is assumed to be part of their illness. If Ms. Chan has a bad night's sleep, this will be brought up at the morning staff meeting, always under the working assumption that it is disease related—but for crying out loud, isn't it obvious that you and I also have a bad night's sleep once in a while? And in response to "sickness," the doctor will give a "treatment," might increase her medication, or might even add a second medication. This problem is worse if something disruptive happens, a quarrel, perhaps, and especially if someone like Wilma Chan is, for example, obsessive about the pedophilia in her family. But I have quarrels too. Who doesn't? In this book, I've been obsessive about the excessive claims of psychiatry, but no one has offered to cool me down with a prescription for clomipramine, let alone forced me to take it against my will.

When ordinary ward behaviours are discussed, there is an implication they are being discussed because something pathological is going on, that the behaviours are a sign of disease and to be recorded in the chart. Limited by the language they've chosen, one designed for biological illness, the staff members forget that all people are strange. Because they use a more wide-ranging language, writers notice the peculiarities of everyday life more clearly than the rest of us: "How lonely and unnatural man is and how deep and well-concealed are his confusions," is how John Cheever put it in his short story "The Leaves, the Lion-Fish, and the Bear." Don't underestimate the coercive power of the hospital meetings—of the disease-language tradition I'm describing. I ran inpatient wards for eight years, and when "problems" arose, the pressure to act was powerful, not because I had to go along with the team, but because I felt the front-line people—the nurses and the clinical assistants—must be right and that my doubts were just silliness. It was the system, the way things were done, and we all felt it was our duty to deal with problems, to take action, to cure people. Yet just like patients, everyone has sleepless nights, most people quarrel, and all of us indulge in our obsessions—the things we're passionate about.

I've called this the sociology of psychiatric hospitals, but usually I call it a language problem. If the chosen language is that of disease, diagnosis, and treatment, the practices I've described are inevitable; if the chosen language is oddness, we will focus differently, on citizenship, human rights, ordinary folly. And it will lead the staff to focus on new issues at the morning staff meeting: "Why is Ms. Chan writing so many emails? How come she's looking after Mr. Grogan all the time? Why is she suddenly reading the Bible? She seems to be worrying about food since Dr. Smith took charge of the ward. Am I right that she's criticizing almost every TV program the others are choosing to watch? Has she neglected her grooming and her makeup recently?"

The analogy in *Cuckoo's Nest* is McMurphy's request that he and the other patients be allowed to watch the World Series on television. In a real psychiatric hospital, the ball games would be on whether or not someone asked. But this film is not about a real hospital; it is a cautionary tale, a warning to the audience that in a hospital, ordinariness can be misread as illness—which is exactly how McMurphy's request is interpreted: everything is mistranslated as a pathological sign.

Rarely will the staff talk seriously to Wilma Chan about her life, her common-law husband, her childhood, her parents. And worst of all, they won't ask her the key question: "How did you get your family and the doctors to put you into the hospital?" In other words, no one will ask the question that might call into question the narrative Ms. Chan first put forward. And if they do, and if she answers, she's unlikely to answer well; instead, she'll blame her doctors, her common-law husband, and others. And that, in fact, is what she did in a second letter written the next day.

March 17, 2014

Dear Dr. Warme

The police picked me up and put me in the hospital in 1995. The doctors said either you can stay here voluntarily or you will be certified. Child welfare forced me to go on meds to get my kids back. I did not know anything about the system. Nobody told me the reasons why I conjured up a thought. Nobody told me about schizophrenia. I know you don't believe in the classification of schizophrenia but there is a whole system that does.

People can easily get that diagnosis and put on meds. Meds is the answer for doctors because of course they don't have to do much work with the patients. They go to school for 6 years and the only thing they have to do is diagnose and hand out pills.

Is there really schizophrenia. Do you believe in all of the research done on it and the experiments. THey do PET scans to find out about the high dopamine. It's too bad I was born in a time like this because it's almost a mark on me the diagnosis.

I dont really think there is a classification of certain people in the world to take meds for the illness. There must be something else. Giving people meds takes away the prosocial behaviour we have as human beings. To talk to and to help. I don't really know if they can find the schizophrenia gene in our DNA.

Thank you for your time.

Sincerely

Wilma Chan

A disappointing answer, but the key issue mustn't be forgotten, the one that matters if she is to become different. What she does in interaction with others *and doesn't reflect upon* is what counts. Every person who works with Wilma Chan should have this issue in mind, trying to steer her toward noticing what she's up to, treating her statements as clues that could enlighten her—not to an answer, but to how enigmatic her life is. Ms. Chan didn't pay serious attention to my suggestion, but I shouldn't give up. Whether or not she thinks about it, her social style, her unhappiness-creating way of understanding the world, is what got her into the hospital. The hospital holding her against her will, giving her drugs she doesn't want, and making her decisions for her are calamities, but no matter how dreadful, they are less important than that she should try to figure out the belief system she has designed for herself, the story that led her to engineer things so the powers that be put her in the hospital. And there's more. How is this a reflection of the rest of her life? Where and when has she done similar things? Why at this time in her life? Whose life is she re-enacting? Don't all of us hear our parents' words come out of our mouths, sometimes the very words we wish we hadn't identified with?

The story of Wilma Chan goes nowhere, and in order to be accurate, the story of Nurse Ratched and McMurphy should also go nowhere; in worlds touched by serious madness, clear endings are rare. My English teachers taught me that all stories have a beginning, a middle, and an end. In the beginning, the characters and setting are introduced, along with a problem; in the middle, the problem escalates and tension, struggle, and conflict ensue as the main character tries to solve it; in the end, there is a resolution. Except the resolution may not be happy, nor is there always a resolution. Adding antidepressants to the water supply won't help.

Cloaked as concern, psychological responses, like the responses of the biologists, can be silly and wrong. When I was a student, one of my supervisors encouraged me with a supposedly memorable line: "Because they are so filled with hatred, so depressed, and so consumed by self-loathing and contempt, working with psychotic patients is difficult. It's very hard to bear." Despite the short-term relief this gave me, it quickly became conspicuous to me that the statement was empty, that these attitudes are no more characteristic of the mad than of anyone else. While some psychotic people hate themselves, many others think well of themselves, are free of depression and contempt. This empty statement is exactly analogous to the empty assumptions that fill psychiatric journals, always interlarded with phrases confirming that these are speculations: "It seems likely that . . ."; "The evidence is closing in . . ." The characteristic of the mad that counts is that their actions are so unconventional that we find them incomprehensible. Apart from momentary relief, a slogan helps neither them nor us. Instead of accepting their behaviour as legitimate, we say that mad life is *illegitimate*.

This makes them targets for our social manipulations and liable to confinement, segregation, and suppression.

At the end of *Madame Bovary*, the heroine takes an overdose of arsenic. Flaubert's description of arsenic poisoning, even today, is more brilliantly evocative than those found in many textbooks of toxicology, and when I was a medical student, Flaubert's description was assigned reading. Flaubert is equally skilled at describing M. Larivière, the consulting doctor who, even though he has no technical skills, visits Emma Bovary. If we psychiatrists must be loyal to our caucus, I suggest keeping to the traditions of our medical ancestry:

> He belonged to that great surgical school created by Bichat—that generation, now vanished, of philosopher-practitioners, who cherished their art with fanatical love and applied it with enthusiasm and sagacity. Everyone in his hospital trembled when he was angry; and his students so revered him that the moment they set up for themselves they imitated him as much as they could... Disdainful of decorations, titles and academies, hospitable, generous, a father to the poor, practicing Christian virtues although an unbeliever, he might have been thought of as a saint if he hadn't been feared as a devil because of the keenness of his mind. His scalpel-sharp glance cut deep into your soul, exposing any lie buried under excuses and reticences. His manner was majestic and genial, conscious as he was of his great gifts and his wealth and the forty years of hard work and blameless living he had behind him.

8

Extracting Sunbeams from Cucumbers

Nothing so needs reforming as other people's habits.
MARK TWAIN, *Pudd'nhead Wilson*, 1894

WHEN WE USE fancy words, we psychiatrists can be fools, like me when I use highfalutin words like *deconstruction*, *Plato*, or *paradigm*, thinking they might impress someone. When a dermatologist says, "You have erythema multiforma"—Latin for funny-shaped red patches on the skin—it is no more helpful than when the psychiatrist says, "You have schizophrenia"—Greek for split mind. We use such words because we are in retreat from the plain truth, using empty diagnostic words as though referring to something real like tuberculosis or an abscess. Violating proper medical practice, many psychiatrists judge their patients' social practices to be normal or pathological, insulting euphemisms that stand in for approval or disapproval. Like literary critics, such psychiatrists have agreed to make judgments: the former make legitimate judgments about artistic performance; thoughtless psychiatrists make judgments about behavioural performance that are *il*legitimate.

Could this be true? Have psychiatrists become social arbiters, moralists who judge their patients' lives? Unfortunately, the answer is yes, a conclusion that makes for unnerving reflections on how many psychiatrists practise. *Unnerving* isn't strong enough; this realization demands a radical rethinking of how psychiatrists (other modern shamans as well) should work and how our predecessors should have worked. The psychiatrist who takes diagnosis seriously has gotten herself into a moralizing and disparaging mess: although she uses the euphemisms *normal* and *abnormal,* words that sound medical, she's actually deciding that certain behaviours are socially acceptable and others not, making a ruling about whether the behaviour is good or bad. Because she wants to be scientific, such a psychiatrist sidesteps these judgmental words, and falls back on words like *disease* and *pathology*, a conclusion nailed down by applying a fancy Greek or Latin word. But the words are wrong. A proper psychiatrist refers to what's going on in ordinary language: *strange*, *tragic*, and *disturbing* are the correct words, important and accurate because they don't insist on pathology.

The person who is crazy, tragic, or stupid is, like anyone else, a private citizen, so in my professional capacity it's none of my business or *any* psychiatrist's business how that person behaves unless he asks for my help. How he behaves is, of course, the business of his family, friends, neighbours, coworkers, and the police, but as a psychiatrist, it's not mine. That I don't like what he is up to and may even worry about it is irrelevant. The psychiatrist should see someone only if asked by the person in question. If a person makes a fool of himself, marries because the planets are in a favourable position, lives on the street, or masturbates in public, the psychiatrist may personally disapprove, but she oughtn't do the closet moralizing called diagnosis. These things are not her affair unless the person in question wants her help. And if the police, the courts, a family member, or another doctor asks the psychiatrist to see the person, she shouldn't agree unless the person himself agrees.

If, on the other hand, the psychiatrist admits that behaviour, even behaviour that makes her uncomfortable, is not a symptom of anything, she'll be better off, less tempted to judge. If a person disturbs the peace or breaks the law, one way or another, civic society, not the psychiatrist, must deal with it. Stanley Fish made this point in the title of his book, *Save the World on Your Own Time*.[1] Understanding this basic point is the

---

1 Stanley Fish, *Save the World on Your Own Time* (New York: Oxford University Press, 2008).

first step in becoming wiser about eccentric and unhappy people, breaking out of the fog we've been in for thousands of years. Yes, thousands.

As long as the psychiatrist is a descriptivist, she is on safe ground; if a *prescriptivist*, she has switched to being a moralist. I say, be a moralist in your private life. Writing this book, for example, is part of my private life and is moralistic. In my office and in the hospital, however, I do my best to stick to describing what I see before my eyes, and carefully rethinking what I see, mostly through the imaginative manipulation of ideas. What's before my eyes is only one thing—a person who tells me his life isn't going well. If he pees on the floor, reveals that he plans to murder his wife, or makes noises that will disturb the patient in the next office, I am still witnessing social practices, but in the face of such dangers, I have to abdicate my psychiatric work temporarily or permanently and act in a socially responsible way. If it's a nuisance problem, I'll try to get the patient to see that he's out to sabotage himself; if it's more than a nuisance (very rare, by the way), I'll refuse to work with him; if it's a crime, I'll report him to the police.

Rather than adjudicating human distress, my job is to do what I can for those who ask for my help, a non-combatant making the best call I can about how to alleviate my patient's suffering. I understand that most of us are at ease with conventional behaviours, but I avoid the problematic word *normal*. I'm cautious because I'm part of a culture that is supposed to respect individuality and uniqueness, a culture that tends to be flexible about weird and unusual behaviour. Even if I don't like them, it's my job to tolerate harmless foibles, even if they are bizarre.

Because I have biases, I can lose my poise and become judgmental, but at my best I study only the unhappiness, oddness, common foolishness, quirkiness, and stupidity that come my way. I'm better at neutrality than I once was, but because my personal craziness is intractable and will regularly cause me to misread things, I have to watch out. That I have veins of craziness should be no surprise—it means I'm ordinary, another human. My madness, subtle and powerful, often catches me unawares, causing me to judge those who, according to my prejudices, don't live the right way. Despite my professional self-reflectiveness, I deceive myself, prefer to think that compared with others, my thinking is reliable. Surely I am prudent, civilized, and normal?

And that is exactly what the fully mad tell us. "Nothing wrong with me," they say.

I'm told that the Japanese word for *different* is the same as the word for *wrong*, which invites a Japanese psychiatrist to say of unusual behaviour, "That behaviour is wrong." In contrast, the German word *Komisch* (as in Komische Oper Berlin) can be translated as *comic* and *fun* or as *strange* and *weird*. Being familiar with the idea that strangeness and fun can be the same thing, German psychiatrists should find it easier than Japanese psychiatrists to understand that oddity need not be seen as pathology.

Yes, the problem is diagnosis. If I apply a disease label, I will think of my patient as ailing, afflicted, passively suffering from some alien thing that has gotten him down, a thing to be got rid of, thereby forgetting that the patient has a hand in everything he does, including the mad part of his life. It's how doctors are trained, and somebody forgot to tell us psychiatrists that when we switch to psychiatric work, all that illness-objectivity stuff has to be forgotten. Doctors are trained to be objective and scientific for good reasons, and in the rest of medicine, the search for abnormalities pays off. Once an abnormality is found, there's a good chance something can be done. But for a psychiatrist, not only is the objective approach useless, it interferes. Looking for an abnormal psychiatric something-or-other promotes earnest searching, but since there's nothing to find, it leads to a futile and unending quest. That's why so many psychiatrists slave away forever, hoping upon hope that the disease, the flaw, the abnormality will go away.

Two thousand years ago, doctors postulated that the bodies of all people contained basic substances, earlier referred to as elements (earth, air, fire, and water), and later referred to as humours (black bile, yellow bile, phlegm, blood). These were considered to be present in a proper balance in all people. Cleopatra agreed. "I am fire and air," she said. "My other elements [the "baser" elements, earth and water] / I give to baser life." A person who was physically ill or psychologically distressed was thought to have an imbalance in these elements or humours and, strangely, in psychiatry nothing has changed: with as little evidence as had the theorists of two thousand years ago, psychiatric patients are said to have abnormal chemicals in their brains. Why do psychiatrists persist in taking the word "disease" literally, thereby failing to realize that in the context of psychiatry, disease is only a figure of speech, a metaphor, just as the ancient elements and humours were metaphors? In the year 2016 I can still say that someone is phlegmatic or melancholic (black bile) and no one takes me literally, assumes that there is really and truly an excess of phlegm or black bile in the person, but the idea of an abnormal chemical is taken very seriously. The psychiatric community suffers from an epidemic of taking things literally, a disease I call *literalis terminalis*.

By not changing their minds when their search for evidence comes up empty-handed, my science-enthralled colleagues are doing what crazy people do—holding onto false beliefs that have no evidential support. I don't say this to mock them, but to dramatize that there is less difference than we usually realize between the thinking of the mad and the rest of us.

I'm not immune. My superstitions are hard for me to notice, just as yours are hard for you to notice. "A very popular error," Nietzsche said, "is having the courage of one's convictions; rather it is a matter of having the courage for an *attack* on one's convictions."[2] But it's a cinch to notice the superstitions in foreign cultures—the Mayans in San Juan Chamula, for example, and the indigenous people of northern Ontario. When we say what is currently fashionable in psychiatric circles, we risk catching the world not in the net of science or truth, but in the net of a problematic tradition.

Unless we are careful, myths can easily trump facts. Everyday observations make it plain that madness and brain abnormality have no necessary connection. At a school for the mentally handicapped, any visitor can see dozens of children with peculiar heads, some with grotesque deformities of the skull, tiny or misshapen. Limited though they are, these children are not mad, crazy, or psychotic. Their obvious physical abnormalities may be shocking and troubling, but even more noticeable is that they act in familiar, childlike ways—not crazy ways. They love their teachers, sing and dance cooperatively, misbehave, giggle, and are regretful when they've been naughty. To insist that

2 Friedrich Nietzsche, *Notebooks*, 1888, 14[159].

brain abnormalities and madness are "obviously" linked is to have not paid attention.

I'm a full-fledged nonconformist, but compared to the mad, I'm a sheep. I have definitely not earned the right to be called a madman. Madmen and madwomen are nonconformists extraordinaire, so different from most people that even I, concerned about demeaning crazy people, am baffled and unnerved. The mad are so extreme that the rest of us won't have it. One or another of the mad will, on one or another occasion, do human things backward:

- Report hearing voices.
- Believe things the rest of us consider preposterous.
- Act wildly disorganized or, contrariwise, hold themselves immobile.
- Think chaotically or with extreme precision.
- Suspect plots or, contrariwise, are utterly credulous.
- React with flattened emotions or, paradoxically, with extreme emotions.

Upon reading this list, it may strike you that something is screwy about the psychiatrist's diagnostic habits: psychiatric diseases can be diagnosed because a certain behaviour is present, and can also be diagnosed on the grounds that it is absent. Unlike other medical diagnoses, psychiatric diagnostic habits look fishy. It doesn't make sense that behavioural signs that contradict each other should lead us to the same diagnostic conclusion. Doctors suspect pneumonia when a patient has a cough and fever, but it would be weird if, on another occasion, the doctor suspected pneumonia because there is *no* cough and fever. The same goes for leukemia. The diagnosis is made according to a primary medical sign—the presence of the cancer cells in the blood, never because of the absence of cancer cells in the blood.

Make no mistake—I'm not saying a few weak researchers ought to be weeded out, drawn, and quartered. I'm making a radical announcement: psychiatry's entire research enterprise is a sham, no different from the research done by the philosophers and scientists on the island of Laputa in Jonathan Swift's *Gulliver's Travels* (1726), the ones busy extracting sunbeams from cucumbers, softening marble for use in pillows, learning how to mix paint by smell, and uncovering political conspiracies by examining the excrement of suspicious persons. Psychiatric research is an example of the human habit satirized by Hermann Hesse in his novel *Magister Ludi* (1943), in which a priestly elite performs a pointless ritual called the glass-bead game.

Medical history is full of such empty practices. As medical students, for example, we were taught the theories of Cesare Lombroso, by then discredited, but several teachers weren't so sure his discreditation was justified. Did these teachers really believe that prostitutes could be identified by taking note of a pathological distribution of their pubic hair? That their appearance was primitive, a sure and dependable sign for identifying them? And when some of us argued that this sounded like nonsense, a highly regarded internist—he'd been brought to the hospital to supervise a wildly popular psychiatric fad called insulin coma treatment—answered that although the specifics may not have been accurate, the general principle—that these people were, as he called them, "throwbacks"—certainly held up. Don't ask me to what they were throwbacks.

Despite millions of dollars spent, thousands of careers launched, and countless awards given, I can't name one *scientific* discovery of a disease or treatment made by a psychiatric researcher, nor do I expect to ever hear about one. I agree that patients are sick in a poetic sense, but I worry about going along with that particular metaphor. Actually, I shouldn't use the mild word *worry*; I should say that I *forbid* the word *sick*. The acceptance of that incorrect word, even as a metaphor, opens the floodgates to the thinking that has been around for thousands of years, gives the thoughtless a chance to mistake metaphoric sickness for real disease and carry on with their malignant stigmatization of people who are unhappy or odd or whose behaviour is bizarre or nervous.

Many psychiatrists risk forgetting to concentrate on the person, the only subject that counts in both the clinic and in the ivory tower. Instead, they focus on the brain and the mind, a decision that forces them, like Descartes, to imagine a magic link exists between the two, saying either that brain is the source of mind, or that mind is the source of brain. As a consequence, they are at risk of making preposterous statements like "His brain is afraid of frogs, is thrilled by the sunset, and has decided to go to Hawaii next winter." Logically, they would then have to accept similarly preposterous statements such as "His mind is manufacturing neurotransmitters, is increasing the frequency of the brain waves in his frontal lobes, and is synthesizing proteins in his amygdala." This malady is commoner than I would have thought. The philosophers Paul and Patricia Churchland are so convinced that brain language should replace intentional language that they converse in what they think is a plausible brain language. Larissa MacFarquhar reports in the *New Yorker* that, having come home from a frustrating faculty meeting, Patricia Churchland spoke to her husband like this:

> Paul, don't speak to me, my serotonin levels have hit bottom, my brain is awash in glucocorticoids, my blood vessels are full of adrenaline, and if it weren't for my endogenous opiates I'd have driven the car into a tree on the way home. My dopamine levels need lifting. Pour me a Chardonnay, and I'll be down in a minute.[3]

It's hard to believe that anyone would take this seriously. Because we all know that brains do only brain things, and people do only people things, it's time for researchers and theoreticians to back off from such nonsense. Patricia Churchland's mood is subject to so many factors that it's preposterous to reduce it to chemicals, especially since her claims are nothing more than that—claims. As always, it's the many people who are terrified of saying "I don't know," even terrified of the word *might*, who make such claims, faith-driven rationalists caught in the trap of scientism. Adrenaline, dopamine, and opiates *might* be involved, but even if they are, so what? There are a billion factors involved, a billion memories, hopes, and fears that will have been stirred up in every day of Patricia Churchland's life. She might (and these are only my imaginings) love her husband, be excited about seeing him, and feel guilty about her marital happiness, a happiness that makes her feel

3 Larissa MacFarquhar, "Two Heads," *New Yorker*, February 12, 2007, p. 59–69.

badly for a less happy sister, colleague, or wife—another *might* that psychiatrists think about.

If a scientist says, "When the brain perceives music, the *X* nucleus is activated and perceives . . ." he's violating the laws of science. Why so? Because the phrase, "the brain perceives music," is silly (I call his the *homuncular fallacy*, the suggestion that the brain or parts of the brain are miniature people). Brains don't perceive anything. Only people perceive, think, and decide. It would be fine if such phrases were thought of as metaphors, but unfortunately the science-enthralled intend these terms to be taken literally. The word *perception* is simply not in the logical universe of brains, but in the logical universe of a person doing something. Yet we are constantly told by researchers—they aren't scientists when they say things like this—that the brain "sends signals," "processes information," and "receives messages." It's people who do these things. Neurons, on the other hand, produce, transmit, and discharge electricity, manufacture and deactivate neurotransmitters, and lots of other physiological things. The stupidity I'm complaining about is analogous to the stupidity I'd be getting into if I tried to use physics to explain why someone is moved by the beauty of a Beethoven string quartet.

Were I to use a metaphor for my friend, for example, say of him that he is my rock, it's unlikely you'd make the linguistic error that leads to psychiatric confusion. You'd neither think he is a gritty, solid lump, nor would you speculate about how he would look at the edge of your flower garden. You'd instantly realize that I find him to be a reliable and loyal friend. But if I said to a diagnostic enthusiast that his wife had roses in her cheeks and that he ought to water them, he'd think I was nuts, as he would if I speculated about the oceanic sources of her coral lips. Were I to insist, he'd indulge the human tendency to concretize metaphors while strongly suspecting I suffered from a disease he'd call schizophrenia. Yet the analogy is exact: roses have to be watered and diseases have to be treated. When a psychiatrist says a patient has split thinking, she's at risk of forgetting that she is talking about an observed social practice, instead believing she's come upon an objective finding, that split thinking is a medical sign that points to a fractured brain function, something actually there.

This is a risk we take—the risk of being misunderstood—every time we use abstract nouns. Even though they refer to things that exist only in thought or theory rather than in matter—*honour, boredom,* or *schizophrenia*, none of which are tangible or concrete—we can't speak completely without them. Yet we can't point to these things; to explain these words, metaphors must be called on. Somehow, we are reassured when we identify something as a (sort of) concrete thing, something (sort of) tangible that can be pinned down. The syntax mistake misses the obvious: abstract nouns don't refer to things; imaginary dumplings won't satisfy your appetite. If we give in to the idea that there are essential truths, we're fundamentalists, as gullible as any cult member. Following Plato, we'd be arguing that real things called truth, justice, and beauty do exist, and if we become Platonic psychiatrists, we'd say real things called social anxiety disorder, schizophrenia, and bipolar illness exist. In contrast, concrete nouns are not abstract, and when we talk about cancer, rheumatoid arthritis, and dengue fever, we are *not* Platonists.

Social practice is the key phrase. Along with curiosity, the phrase *social practice* should inform everything the psychiatrist thinks about—for two reasons. First, taking note of social practices is simpler, more obvious, and far more accurate than saying there is a "something" called disease that invisibly lies behind the social practice (to tell the truth, those who make this error don't even notice that what they are making a diagnosis about is a social practice) and assumed to be real. Description, although imperfect, keeps us from going astray. Phrases like *split mind* and *brain dysfunction* are actually conclusions derived out of thin air, close kin to wild conclusions like cosmic influence and demon possession. Because they're not descriptive, they lead us into la-la land. The second great value of the term *social practice* is that it nails down the fact that the only thing we psychiatrists ever see in our patients is their interaction with other people, that when we study someone, we aren't studying him in isolation, that we must use a field theory. In parallel with quantum theory, we keep—or ought to keep—uppermost in our minds that a person exists only as part of an ensemble. When we psychiatrists think about a patient, we're dealing with a linked phenomenon, an interpersonal dynamic, a patient-psychiatrist singularity. Another way of saying this is that instead of paying attention to the *things* referred to by a word, we should attend to the use made of the word, the *behaviour* being pointed to by words like *depression* and *schizophrenia*.

A psychiatric disorder is diagnosed by noting the patient's statements, his descriptions of what he is doing and experiencing and, to a lesser extent, descriptive statements made by other observers. But the psychiatrist shouldn't take her patient's words at face value; her job is to study how she and her patient interact and when she can, how the patient interacts with others. She shouldn't, for example, believe it when her patient says his brain is damaged by poisons. But when a psychiatrist talks about abnormal brain chemicals, she's done that very thing: fallen into the trap of believing her patient's crazy thoughts. Because it may be exactly what the patient wants to get going, there's also no point in arguing. What she ought to do is to stay out of the fray and to confine herself to simply observing: "Hmm, once again it's bad things happening to you and your brain, once again you as the loser. Why the devil is it so important to you to always think of yourself as losing out and of your brain as damaged?"

The psychiatric community insists otherwise, that we are to take the patient's words to be signs of disease. The diagnosis is then made by noting that the person fits certain pre-established criteria—nowadays, the DSM-5 criteria I mentioned in chapter 4—something that can be done with a modest measure of reliability. But this "reliability" is not confirmed by correlating the psychiatrist's diagnoses with objective, biological pathology; it means only that a number of people use the same language for a person's behaviour. This "reliability" can convince a psychiatrist that the project of discovering diseases is legitimate. But reliability has nothing to do with validity. The obvious example is that any set of behaviours, lumped together, can be called a disease, then reliably "diagnosed" by an examiner. Normal, foolish, shy, charmer, athlete, mechanic, and intellectual—any way of life that can be imagined can be lumped together this way. Kendra, who helps me out at my cottage, told me that she, too, suffers from a psychiatric disorder. "Please get Windex for next week because I'm 'window-anal,'" she said. This disorder can, of course, be reliably diagnosed, but despite her claim, I doubt that her self-diagnosis is *valid*.

Only the study of social practices pays off. If an Indian-Canadian man phones his mother in Bombay and asks her advice about the mortgage he is taking on, his wife interprets this as ordinary and socially fitting; if a Canadian man does the same, his wife may well interpret his actions differently, fearing this means he's a momma's boy. In contrast, a crushing pain behind the sternum suggests heart attack, a real disease, irrespective of culture. Traits and surface behaviours are unique to individuals, so it's useless to think we could ever tally, weigh, or measure them; there is no pathology or health standard.

If, having worked with me, the patient joins in and becomes an artistic observer of his own ways, I have to be careful about being impressed and complimentary. All that can honestly be said is that, on a particular day, the patient thought and talked in this way or that. For sure it would be stupid to say that the patient had changed for the better. Many patients would disagree, sure that their adoption of an aesthetic view of themselves is a worthwhile change, but the psychiatrist restrains her enthusiasm, wants only to think further about things, even when patients start to do what the psychiatrist has been doing: pondering their own speeches, watching their own behaviour, becoming their own thoughtful critics—"cured," so to speak. The disease of which they've been cured? Ordinary folly, self-ruinous behaviours, and idiocies just like their psychiatrist's.

PART THREE

PSYCHOTHERAPY ON THE COUCH

9

The Maiden-in-Distress Complex

As a man is, so he sees.
WILLIAM BLAKE

I'M HAVING COFFEE on the patio of the Hotel de Cortés in Mexico City, a small hotel that was once a monastery. At the next table are a woman and her daughter, the girl about sixteen with white teeth and tender brown arms. The youngster gives a small cough, and I glance over. The girl notices my glance and drops her eyes. The mother has also noticed and a shadow flits across her face. She suspects I'm a lecher, but the truth is different; I'm a romantic and, in my mind, the potentially lecherous scene is cleaned up: *The girl is Mimi in* La Bohème, I was thinking, *doomed, a waif with a tubercular cough, in need. Not only am I a doctor, I am Rodolfo, the impoverished writer who will save her.*

It's a scene so slight that only by watching closely would one notice that the girl, polite and innocent, is not innocent after all—she knows that men are interested. And the mother too knows that her daughter now has a place at the centre of the heterosexual stage. Although it points at something common and real, I don't want to admit that my line of thought is a platitude—the dashing hero, destined to save the girl, sweeps her off her feet and teaches her about love and passion and life and truth and sex, transforming her. Even though at my age I've used up most of my allotted time, she will, in this fancy, never forget me. The girl and I have been transformed into operatic characters: rather than a youngster with a trivial cough, she is an ill and dying heroine; instead of personifying decrepitude, I am a dashing hero. It's the favourite story of all time: the heroic man (James Bond, Superman, Rudolph Valentino) will save the maiden in distress (Snow White, Lois Lane, Tess of the d'Urbervilles).

At a meeting of supervisors, we all agreed that when the doctor is a man—especially obvious in students—and the patient is a woman, the *La Bohème* configuration is always smouldering in the background—or out in the open. As you have seen, I am as ready as anyone else to live out the Rodolfo and Mimi scenario, to move into action when I hear a young girl's cough—to see a woman as frail. In this traditional story, a woman patient decides it's her destiny to be saved by her wonderful doctor—except isn't this a trap, a fairy tale? Does it make sense for a psychiatrist to repeat what goes on everywhere else? I call it the maiden-in-distress complex.

KENNETH EUSTON WAS a pal of mine, a fellow student at the Menninger Clinic in Topeka, Kansas. Originally from Canterbury in England, he was a graduate of Guy's Hospital medical school in London and already a Member of the Royal College of Physicians, at that time a prerequisite for studying psychiatry in the United Kingdom. Ken had come to the United States because he was interested in psychoanalysis, very different from the phenomenological focus of British training programs. Like me, Ken had chosen to do his first two years of psychiatric training in Topeka because of Karl Menninger, then the best-known psychiatrist in the world. Just before coming to Topeka, Ken had spent a few months in Princeton, New Jersey, in order to study under the philosopher Walter Kaufmann, the world-famous Nietzsche scholar at Princeton. Both Kaufmann and Menninger were intellectual superstars, and Ken was determined to be in contact with world-class teachers. While in Topeka, Ken worked intensively with a psychotherapy case, supervised by Elise Workman, a tough and demanding teacher, sought after by many students but avoided by those nervous about criticism. When he discussed the patient at our weekly case conference, Ken turned out to have a formidable mind, talking like someone with years of experience.

Everyone loved Ken. He was kind and intelligent, worked hard and, without being pedantic, obscure, or pretentious, used philosophical insights when he spoke up at meetings. Despite a gentle nature, he did speak up, both at small case conferences and at larger meetings, the place where senior teachers did most of the talking. His influence changed our small local case conferences; we practical-minded psychiatrists were stimulated to think and discuss things more deeply when he drew our attention to the ideas of Ludwig Wittgenstein, Gilbert Ryle, Friedrich Nietzsche, and Clifford Geertz—scholars who, rather than theorizing abstractly, talked and wrote about what people actually do—and how these ideas could sharpen our thinking.

One day, while Ken and I were having lunch, he told me that the year before he came to Topeka, he'd broken up with his girlfriend of long standing in his hometown of Canterbury. She'd sent him an ominous note and he'd rushed to her digs, put a ladder against the house, and gone in through the window. She had killed herself and, obviously, Ken was still feeling guilty.

After two years in Topeka, Ken moved back to London, where he finished his training. A year or so later, I heard he'd written about the case he'd treated while in Topeka, a book that had become a minor bestseller. The case had had a good outcome, so the book was a sort of happy-ending story. I wasn't surprised because I'd seen Ken's clear-thinking style when he'd spoken at case conferences during our training together. When I told Elise Workman Ken had written a book about the successful outcome of the case, instead of being pleased, she opened her eyes wide and blurted, "What?"

What a crab, I thought.

A few years after leaving Topeka, Ken returned for a visit on his way to a meeting in Chicago. Elise, Ken, and I had dinner. Elise spoke to him harshly. "I've read your book. Don't you remember what we talked about when we met for supervision? It was always the same thing. Your patient had repeatedly screwed up her life by falling in love with men who didn't suit her—she idealized them and saw them as heroes and then had her heart broken. That's why she came to see you. You saw her only about twenty times, Ken, yet in the book you suggest that you saved her, changed her life. But for Christ's sake, when the treatment stopped because you were going back to England, she was blindly idealizing *you* and turning *you* into a hero—nothing had changed except that the same self-destructive thing she always did, she was doing with you. Don't you remember we talked about this repeatedly, how worried we were that her madness was happening again with you, and that you wouldn't have time to analyze it properly before you left? What were you thinking when you wrote the book?"

Ken was stunned, and I was taken aback by Elise's bluntness. But she was determined to get her point across. When she had responded crankily to the news that Ken had written a book about his case, I'd thought she was just being her usual critical self, but now I understood. A well-known human madness had appeared in Ken's patient, and he had transformed this into an inspirational story of love, cure, salvation. And, I thought, the suicide of Ken's girlfriend back in Canterbury was also in the mix. Later, Ken and I corresponded about what had happened. He understood what Elise had said and had become depressed, very depressed. It wasn't just embarrassment over a professional misstep; my memory is that Ken's depression lasted for several years.

Elise hadn't spoken to Ken properly. Instead of scolding him, she'd have gotten further by reminding him of *La Bohème*, of Mimi and her little cough, of Eliza Doolittle, and of countless other mythological versions of these stories—Ariadne, Andromeda, Brünnhilde, all maidens who need rescuing. If, instead of scolding, she had tempted him to try out a different language when he thought about cases, if she'd spoken sympathetically, told him that every one of us has rescue fantasies, he might have listened. She might have said, "God help us if we think we can really and truly pull off such rescues." Then she could have told Ken to give himself a little pinch whenever he was tempted to think he was Prince Charming or Mother Teresa. She might even have made a joke: "Ken, if you find yourself getting into this kind of thing again, just pop over the pond from England and I can give you a quick pinch."

In London, Ken organized a Nietzsche study group in which he and some other psychiatrists joined up with some philosophers to discuss how, with her patient, the psychiatrist examines moral dilemmas and self-deceptions just as Nietzsche did. Since he knew I was also interested in this topic, when I visited London a few years later, Ken introduced me to a supposed Nietzsche expert whose name I can't recall. I hoped we'd have a good discussion about truth and its elusiveness, especially the idea that truth and language go hand in hand. When we got to Ken's place, as soon as the introductions were over, this so-called expert narrowed his eyes, glowered at me, and demanded, "Who are the three most important philosophers of the twentieth century?"

Taken aback, I mumbled something incoherent, probably mentioning Wittgenstein and Nietzsche.

"Wrong," announced this ass. "The three most important philosophers of the twentieth century are the early Nietzsche, the middle Nietzsche, and the late Nietzsche." Who the hell ever heard of Nietzsche divided into eras? It's not even a good joke. For the rest of the evening, nothing came out the fool's mouth but arbitrary pronouncements.

Still in London and over drinks in Ken's flat, I chatted with a woman who was a member of the seminar study group that Ken had set up. "Ken and I are writing a book," she said. "I was his patient and we're writing up what happened in the therapy." Oh my God. I wasn't sure I wanted to hear about this. Writing another book about a case, this time *with* the patient, with a one-time patient, didn't sound like a good idea.

A few months later—I was living in my hometown of Toronto by then—I received a letter from another friend in London who also knew Ken, a gossipy, wait-till-you-hear-this letter: "Something has happened to Ken. He was writing a book with a patient and they've gotten into a disagreement, bad enough that he's in trouble with his professional association, the General Medical Council." The letter didn't explain or give details about the scandal, so my imagination had a field day. Like everyone, I can't resist juicy scandal, so my reaction to this news was mixed: I was worried about Ken, I was self-righteously indignant at his grandiosity, and I loved the potential wickedness of the scandal. I also had fantasies about what had happened—maybe they'd had an affair, Ken living out the prince and the maiden-in-distress complex again.

I could only imagine that Ken had been sure he knew the cure, the magic treatment. Like healers throughout the millennia, most of us fall into that trap for a while, keen to think we've found a substantial, honest-to-God, not-just-symbolic cure for madness. Frankly, I should use stronger words, language that makes it clear that like many before me (and I don't often admit this), I want to be a hero, a champion, the person who inspires, who finally, once and for all, leads people to Jerusalem, to a finer life, to maturity, wisdom, and prosperity, new citizens of the communities of the future. Let's face it—I want to be God.

But even God failed. More than two thousand years ago, fed up with the ancient Israelites (the Israelites, like modern Jews, and like Alvy Singer's family in the film *Annie Hall*, were noisy and squabbled too much) and being addicted to problem solving just like modern psychiatrists, God decided to change things. First, he decided that the behavioural signals given off by the Jews were evidence that they had a disease, so he applied a diagnosis: "squabbling disorder, cultural type, chronic and severe, characterized by noisiness and arguments over trivialities, sometimes viewed as charming, but ultimately self-defeating and definitely pathological." Once he had a diagnosis, God was ready for therapeutic action, something dramatic, so he raped a virgin Jewess by the name of Mary. Surprisingly, this rape led to something important: Christianity, an obedient rather than a squabbling religion (at least initially), was born. Mary had conceived immaculately, and the world was transformed.

But God's transformation of Judaism into Christianity inspired neither a cure nor a rehabilitation of the world. Despite what he had hoped for, his intervention with the squabbling Jews didn't work. Ken's transformation of dependent patients into admirers and devotees also didn't work; instead, his interventions, if they accomplished anything at all, created dependency and sexual longing. Like the many psychiatrists enamoured of ecstasy and magic, God had thought he could transfigure the world.

Despite God's failure, maybe there *are* tricks that work. If you feel guilty because you've hurt your friend's feelings, soothe yourself with a dose of self-scolding; if hubby forgets your wedding anniversary, you'll feel better if you banish him, put him under the bed for the night. Of course, guilt and hurt feelings aren't diseases, so these psychological tricks aren't real cures, either. The same goes for a psychiatric patient: since there's not a scrap of evidence that anxiety, despondency, and extreme oddity are diseases, it's moot whether psychiatrists' favourite methods—drugs, talking, electric shocks—cure him. But these methods *do* achieve something, sometimes as a placebo effect and sometimes because the patient is helped to rethink how he lives his life.

I'M BEING OBSESSIVELY critical of Ken, so it's time to do some thinking. Whether I like it or not, I'm part of the problem, mostly because of my allegiance to the second of psychiatry's major ideologies, not biology, but psychoanalysis. Freud's theories have affected us all, but during a major part of the twentieth century, psychiatry was more than affected: psychoanalysis dominated Western psychiatry, most of all in the United States. Before Freud, academic psychiatrists focused on identifying and classifying mental diseases and speculating about the causes of mental disorders, but once Freud suggested that mental diseases could be treated and cured, his ideas became a firestorm that consumed Western psychiatry. The centrepiece of his thinking was the unconscious, the idea that all of us, including psychiatrists and psychiatric patients, must deal with a variety of unconscious torments. Every person is inspired to live in a way designed to fend off or manage these stresses and anxieties. Freud's original observations did not focus on ways in which people lived, but on *symptoms* designed to fend off or manage these tensions. What I've called the patient's *way of living* includes those symptoms as well as his character style, his ideological preferences, and his theories about how life is best lived. Later, because no way of life is unique and practised by only one person, I'll say he has signed up with a tribe, an "interpretive community," or better, a number of interpretive communities.

In building his theory, Freud used a bad philosophical model—Aristotelian mechanics. His ego, id, superego, and drives model was a sort of machine, ill suited to issues of human behaviour. I'd rather stick to a theory that says it in a way analogous to this: if I forcefully think red, red, red, I can't think of its complementary colour green; if I think lose, lose, lose, I can't think of winning; if I concentrate on being pure and clean, holy and sacred, I need never think of myself as a sexy, dirty pig; if I devote my life to helping the poor, I'll never be troubled by thinking myself greedy; if I'm bizarre and crazy, I'll never have to take on the problems of being a responsible citizen. This model—I might call it structuralism, as is often preferred by European psychiatrists and linguists, but it is also semiology, the theory of signs. Because every patient is, for me, a foreign culture, I'm inclined to think of myself as a sort of anthropologist, so I was pleased when a French student, after spending a year of training in Toronto before returning to Paris, sent me a postcard. "It's such a relief to be back here," she wrote. "In the corridors of the hospital, I hear people talking: '*Le désir, la demande, la demande impérative.*'" (That is to say, a *demand impérative* is experienced lest a different and more worrisome *demand impérative* show its face.)

Here's how we humans set up such ways of living, such *observable* ways of living: when you fear that the bogeyman is under your bed, in a flurry of cleverness, you tell yourself it's just the wind. Wind, wind, wind is easier to live with than the bogeyman, bogeyman, bogeyman. You might also say that the sound under your bed is your imagination, a creaky board, or an undigested bit of Skippy peanut butter, metaphors that replace the unwelcome bogeyman. All of us design for ourselves certain ways of life, adopt certain styles, use certain analogies, ideologies, and especially opposites (in our offices we psychiatrists call them symptoms, diseases, or personality disorders) that make it easier to live with our fantastic, born-in-childhood fears—the psychiatric patient's warded-off bogeyman equivalents.

The self-comforting cover story or way of life is the only thing the psychiatrist sees. But the psychiatrist is trying to untangle things that are more substantial, her patient's *character*, the deeply embedded style that infuses his every thought and every behaviour. Even awful things like conscious anxiety and conscious depression are understood to be modes of thinking that cleverly ward off demons, unconscious demons that seem worse than the anxiety or depression the patient is aware of. Hysterics do the same: horrible and disfiguring paralyses, blindness, and fits are psychologically based infirmities that force out of the mind issues that are deemed to be even worse than paralyses, blindness, and fits. The psychiatrist is after *personal* ideologies, not the religious, political, and social ideologies of everyday life.

In each of the following points, the statement from the patient is the unconscious issue or dread, and in square brackets is what's conscious, the behavioural/ideological compromise:

- "From the way people react to me, I suspect I'm a real cutie-pie, get away with murder with Mom and Dad, which is also fun because there's an exciting sexual side to it. But because I'm so appealing to everyone, it's clear that other people in the family are overshadowed by me, which disturbs them—and it's my fault. In the interest of everyone's well-being, it's best that I curb myself, banish charm and sex from my life except in a watered-down way. If it turns out I do become sexually alive, I'll make sure that my relationships always end in disaster." [Women: develop conversion hysteria, disabling physical ailments. Men: become wimps, weaklings, sissies.]
- "I have a feeling that my family and friends find me a useless bore, think of me as a pathetic flop. To hell with that. I'm going to make sure that I always look potent and sexy." [Women: become erotically tantalizing, provocative, domineering. Men: become bullies, Lotharios, braggarts.]
- "This artistic side of me means that I'm smarter and more creative than everyone else in the family. It reminds them of how mediocre they are, a nasty scenario I really don't like. I'll fix this by adopting a modest low profile." [Either sex: become a hermit-philosopher, drink too much, stay unmarried, take on a modest job.]

Formulated as a hypothesis, here is how this psychological strategy looks:

All people, especially as children, are troubled by things they think might be dangerous within themselves (petty crimes, envy, hatred, lust, popularity, beauty, achievement, and so on), things they undo in their adult life by seizing on one of the various roles available in our culture (genius, psychiatrist, thief, loser, discarder of women, miser, hermit, traveller, health food fanatic—or a psychiatric symptom). The role they've chosen, when studied in the psychiatrist's office, can be seen to obscure dangerous scenarios they'd once dreamed up about themselves. Note that trauma and bad parenting aren't central to the theory.

Of course, these are caricatures and generalizations. The ideologies of real people are unique, subtle, and much more imaginative, but you get the idea—it's Freud's great redescription of human life, the notion of the unconscious. The psychoanalytic cure aims to unearth such issues, untangle them, and carefully, politely, and imaginatively insist on many points of view (Nietzsche: "Truth is a mobile army of metaphors") that stand against the fixed point of view the patient has ensnared himself in. The many points of view are interpretations or metaphors that the psychiatrist injects into the conversation, *insists* on injecting into the conversation. Since it's common to talk of ideas being "played off" one another, why do I say *insist*? Well, because Hegel's ideas are one of the underpinnings of Freud's idea of change. Hegel argued that when a person puts forward a *thesis*, another person can put forward an *antithesis*, a struggle more forceful than is implied by "played off." Out of this competition of ideas comes something new, a *synthesis*. In other words, the patient puts forward his ideology, the psychiatrist puts forward a series of counter-ideologies, and the result is a synthesis, something new, a change. There's not much for the patient to argue against because the psychiatrist doesn't argue on behalf of a particular point of view. One minute she mentions the importance of easing up, the next minute introduces the idea of attack, resolve, determination—only to reverse fields again and speak of sensuality and poetry. The patient, a bit off balance, comes face to face with his pedestrian repetitiousness.

The unconscious still burbles away, unending and relentless, even though its existence as a hard fact is open to doubt. The psychiatrist talks about the unconscious only in spurts of metaphor. What else could she do? The "unconscious" doesn't exist in any substantial physical or mental sense; rather, it's a word that refers to vaguely sensed terrors, to an abyss of envy, lust, greed, vanities—mental complexes, if you like—that live on forever because they are nothing more than potential actions and thoughts. Were she to think of the unconscious as a container with real things in it, the psychiatrist would be inventing demons as spurious as the abnormal chemicals invented by biological psychiatrists. She'd also be falling into the trap of determinism, thinking that Oedipus complexes, narcissistic complexes, and Electra complexes "cause" certain behaviours—just as biologists say imaginary chemicals "cause" certain behaviours. The proper use of terms such as the Electra complex is to call them analogies. A psychiatrist might say, "Well, Mr. Glickson, when you tell stories about the smells you noticed in the bathroom after your mother had been in there, it's analogous to the

Oedipus story, something about intimate secrets about your mother that you felt uneasy about. We can speculate that, like Prince Oedipus, you were shocked. Oedipus's shock was when he discovered that he had inadvertently married his mother." The psychiatrist focuses on what she sees in front of her eyes and makes comparisons, devises interesting images that illuminate the patient's style—his defensive strategies and manoeuvres. Once the patient notices that his ways are ill-chosen attempts at self-reassurance—with an emphasis on *ill-chosen*—things won't be the same; instead, different ways and ideas will take over, this time formulated by an adult, not by a frightened child.

Informed psychoanalysts (note that most psychoanalysts are psychiatrists who later train as psychoanalysts, although a smaller number are psychologists, educators, sociologists, who also pursue psychoanalytic training *after* they have their advanced degree) should be able to teach biological psychiatrists how to stay scientific, except for the inconvenient fact that psychoanalysts commonly make the same error as the biologists. Like biologists who believe that imaginary chemicals and brain abnormalities really exist in their patients' bodies, these psychoanalysts believe that imaginary Oedipus complexes, fixations, drives, bad experiences with parents, weak egos, and harsh superegos really exist. Because he hoped to make his theories scientific, Freud himself fell into that trap, trying to use objectivity to discover "abnormal" things—things I posit are just different points on the scale of what's normal.

When he wrote about cases, Freud didn't make this mistake, didn't use such fictions. On a few occasions he improved his theoretical arguments by asserting that in the end, the unconscious is composed of the "primal repressed"—that is to say, is something never accessible to us. He'd have been better off had he said this plainly—that the unconscious, in a literal sense, doesn't exist. Freud is in very good form and interesting in chapter 2 of *The Interpretation of Dreams*, the section called "The Analysis of a Specimen Dream" (also known as "The Dream of Irma's Injection").[1] It is one of Freud's own dreams, and in his report he makes

---

1 Sigmund Freud. "The Interpretation of Dreams," *The Standard Edition of the Complete Psychological Works of Sigmund Freud*, Vol. 4 (London: The Hogarth Press, 1953): chapter II, p. 96.

no reference to mental "things." My conclusion: both biologically and psychologically oriented psychiatrists would be better off concentrating on what's before their eyes.

DESPITE MYSELF, IT'S clear that rather than merely having a healthy interest in an important theory, I'm ideologically devoted to Freud's major idea of the unconscious (I'm less vulnerable to Freud's weak ideas, of which there are plenty). Too excited by the theory of the unconscious, I forget that theories aren't precious, and they certainly aren't things; there's no finger-thumb reality (self-explanatory philosopher jargon) that lies behind a theory. Theories are tools for thinking and experimenting, and they end up being good for some things and useless for others. My pliers are good for cutting wire but useless for cutting the veal chop on my dinner plate. If I buy into a theory unreservedly, I've joined the ranks of the superstitious, no different from the colleagues I complain about. Besides, if I'm out to deconstruct the ideologies of my patients, surely that deconstructive attitude applies to me as well; if I'm *caught up* in psychoanalysis rather than being merely *interested* in it, not only am I contradicting the intent of the theory, I'm blinkering myself in my work with patients.

But I like Freud's psychoanalytic theory of the unconscious (I'm doing better; "like" is safer than "ideologically devoted to"), including its strange commitment to never being committed to an ideology. I'm determined to deconstruct all thoughts and actions of my patients, whether they cause trouble for my patients or not. I aim to be thorough, to hold nothing sacred or true, although I inevitably have a bias toward tackling moral dilemmas that strike me as self-sabotaging. That analytic bent kindles my crankiness with my colleague Ken—and with lots of other people too. I'm annoyed that, rather than analyzing the maiden-in-distress complex and doing as much self-examination as he might have, Ken indulged these things. A patient feels great if he can admire his psychiatrist, but the psychiatrist might get further by helping the patient to re-examine each of his torments and triumphs. It's also not just me—the whole psychoanalytic tribe belittles treatments that don't analyze deeply. Scornfully, we call Ken's successes "transference cures"—fake cures, in other words. Our way, we say, is the "real" treatment: unravel every ideology, belief, habit, and taste—indeed, every breath. A number of artists I've known have said that because of the habit of analyzing everything, they avoid psychoanalysis, concerned that it will unravel everything, including their talent.

To be in psychoanalysis is a piece of good luck for those who experience it, a chance for change, and a chance to experience first-hand an important way of thinking. And that's what it is—a vital contribution to how we think about human life. Psychoanalysis influenced psychiatrists to do psychotherapy, which, in turn, led to the tremendous public interest in psychotherapy. Critical as I am, I wince at naïve distortions of psychoanalysis, even though I try to be sensible and settle for the most important thing: *psychiatry (usually) recognizes that it is important for our patients to have a chance to talk to a doctor.* Most psychoanalysts would differ on this point and say that *it is important for our patients to discover the unconscious motives for why they live and think the way they do.* I agree with both groups. However, dozens of psychotherapies have come and gone during my career, most designed to avoid the length and cost of traditional psychoanalysis. Instead of shortening psychotherapeutic treatments, I suggest something else: every time a psychiatrist talks to a patient, she should speak in a psychoanalytically informed way, be it a five-minute exchange in a corridor or on the phone, or twenty regularly scheduled meetings. Why not use valuable knowledge whenever she can?

10
Change

Dear is Plato, but dearer still is truth.
ARISTOTLE

We possess art lest we perish of the truth.
NIETZSCHE

I LIKE ARISTOTLE'S APHORISM. Reading it, like any and every event, changed me just a bit. At minimum it will become a small memory, so it's safe to say that even if small, change is possible. But Aristotle's aphorism is nothing more than a well-put platitude, not up to the job of inducing change that matters. Nietzsche's aphorism also changed me, and because it made me think a little, the change it induced in me, although still slight, was more substantial. In addition to having art lest we perish of the truth, the aphorism makes me realize that we possess psychiatry lest we perish of the truth, we possess love lest we perish of the truth, and we possess war lest we perish of the truth. But if I look at the two aphorisms together, the effect on me and the change they induce is more definite: considered together, the aphorisms contradict each other, stir me up, no longer add up to a platitude—and force me to think. Right this minute, the two aphorisms remind me of something about myself, that I overestimate the value of "truth," or, at my most dogmatic, that I believe in "truth at all costs." One aphorism leads to change; two aphorisms pressure me to think carefully. *Maybe it doesn't make sense to tell the woman on the subway train the truth, that her legs are beautiful; maybe I should think twice before I mock the Prophet Mohammed by way of a cartoon; maybe, if I'm introduced to Queen Elizabeth II, there's no need to tell her that her clothes are dowdy.*

Truthfulness is tricky.

Since my job is to help people to change, and because platitudes play only a small role in change (trivialities can lead to change—a broken tooth, a song, a bonus at work—but rarely durable change), I avoid them when I can. But it's hard. In day-to-day life we live according to long lists of platitudes, their purpose being to encourage us to behave conventionally, reassure us that we are citizens in good standing, still linked with our community. They calm things down and keep our cultural systems going. What's ordinarily done is to help a troubled person fit in with the interpretive communities of which he is a member, the tribes and solidarities in which he lives, the worlds where people marry, have children, and eat Tim Horton's donuts, worlds that contain stable categories of thinking and behaving. Most of us believe in the ways of that world. If I'm talking to a patient, I know he will already have given himself repeated pep talks that are in keeping with this everyday life, platitudes his family and friends will also have recommended. But when ordinary helpfulness doesn't work, there's no payoff if the psychiatrist does the same thing as friends and family; psychiatrists exist precisely for those times when giving platitudinous reassurance hasn't worked. There's also no payoff in advising someone that *most* people do such-and-so.

By "interpretive community," I mean something complicated, even if most of us effortlessly negotiate our own interpretive communities, our tribes. All of us identify with many such communities, sometimes quietly, sometimes noisily:

- Jewish, Christian, Muslim, Buddhist, and their various subcategories
- black, white, Asian, indigenous, and their typical attitudes and habits
- conservative, liberal, socialist, communist, anarchist, pacifist, revolutionary, fascist
- butcher, baker, candlestick maker, jobless, CEO, bootlegger, thief

- sexy, sexless, feminist, passive, bold, lover, humorous, boring, flashy, braggart, meek
- artist, tone-deaf, observer, creator, self-promoter, hermit, misogynist, terrorist
- handsome, beautiful, ordinary, ugly
- lower class, middle class, upper class, old money, new money, white trash, Johnny-come-lately

All of us identify with hosts of categories, communities of people who interpret the world the way we do, interpretive communities, in other words. Bizarre, evil, or admirable, each is opted for by some. Here is a personal example: I subscribe to the *New York Review of Books* and faithfully read it every two weeks. I don't learn much—I already know and agree with the opinions I'm reading—but the magazine is a scripture to me, tells me that I belong to the tribe of people called liberal intellectuals. The familiar incantations on the pages of the magazine reassure me that I am who I think I am. My modest-sized diesel-engine car also reassures me, sustains a certain image I have of myself, as does my wristwatch, a stainless-steel Rolex Submariner I've had for forty-five years. Tribal affiliations can be obvious but are also to be sniffed out in small details. Interpretive communities provide ways of thinking that the patient has arranged for himself, ways that in a particular person are extraordinarily complicated, even as they are part of a general community of styles and values.

Rather than getting to the truth, what people believe in is an option, a link with a like-minded community. While all of us are sure of our favourite beliefs, in fact, none of these loyalties is correct. The truth is actually ugly news, especially when it includes wholesale skepticism about our inner worlds, a reminder that our memories are biased, parochial, and self-serving. Even memories that make us look bad serve our own purposes. Worst and hardest is to be skeptical of ourselves. Because most of us are inveterate blamers, we're adroit at hanging on to our memories of others having been stupid and nasty toward us, enamoured of finding fault with others. But pointing out such things is what we deconstructionist psychiatrists are up to, not noisily, not evangelically, but quietly, mildly, with humour, nostalgia, regret, and—most important—with fascination at the peculiarity of our patients' and our own minds.

Here are a few more tribes, interpretive communities, whose truths many of us believe in: always gentle and kind, always tough and determined, always refined and dignified, eternally a victim needing rescue, a continual rescuer, a student of human behaviour, a wet blanket, a derelict, a leader, a fool, the wealthy, or the zealously religious. And to make this pertinent to psychiatry, there is depression (low opinion of oneself, self-insulting talk—"I've wrecked my family's life"; "I'm a lazy good-for-nothing"), extreme craziness ("My cell phone is sending my confidential information to my boss"; "The television is telling me to hurt someone"), or anxiety ("If I'm introduced to this person, I will faint, my voice will be paralyzed, I'll have to rush out of the living room in clear sight of all the guests"). To completely unravel someone's tribal affiliations is impossible, but that's what the psychiatrist is out to do. She aims to destabilize the patient's interpretive world and his madness world—the same thing—so he will be freer to follow new ways. She does this by repeatedly showing him what he does, by being highly curious about these ways, and by linking them with a profusion of analogous behaviours in his current life and his history. Because these behaviours are subtly different and disguised, the patient does not always immediately recognize them. And sometimes they are wilfully not seen because, as one patient said, he gets a mind-cramp when about to see a new link. These self-sabotaging behaviours point to the tribes with which the patient has aligned himself, having decided that his decision that living according to the interpretive communities called *a*, *b*, and *c* is best.

Serious change depends on the patient changing how he thinks, requires that he *try out novel ways of thinking, sign on with new interpretive communities, acquire new tribal affiliations, identify with new solidarities*. Because the psychiatrist doesn't know better than anyone else how the patient should live his life, she doesn't advocate a particular set of convictions for the patient to sign on with—except that, without ever trying to sell it, she is a model of a particular set of convictions: deconstructive, analytic, interpretive, postmodern. Theoretically, she has no opinion on whether the patient should become prime minister, revolutionary, philosopher, monk, hermit, or a suicide: on that score, she is neutral. But no matter how hard she tries to be neutral, her personal agendas will be obvious to the patient. About that, little can be done.

The psychiatrist is a saboteur; she interferes with stale beliefs that, before he met her, her patient held to be truths he *had* to live by. Always in the back of her mind is the idea that she wants to unravel everything her patient has ever believed in, to wipe the slate clean. She wants to persuade him that, most importantly, the interpretive communities he has identified with do not have the inside track on truth, beauty, or duty, and second, that she, his psychiatrist, embodies a different interpretive community, one he has probably not thought about before but may be interested in. That interpretive community is not fascism, Christianity, "getting with the program," anarchy, or getting rich; rather, it's vague and confusing.

The collapse of absolute monarchies and dictatorships and the loss of absolute belief in God have meant that the truth no longer comes down from above and that, more than we once did, people think for themselves and aren't so sure about gods and established rituals. And that's what modernism is—new thinking is permissible, even if some people hate it. This confusing, deconstructive attitude became popular in the late nineteenth and early twentieth centuries. Friedrich Nietzsche and Sigmund Freud (clear writers, easy to read) were among the earliest members of this interpretive community, followed by people like Martin Heidegger and Jacques Lacan (impossible to read—I've given up), Ludwig Wittgenstein and Jacques Derrida (hard to read), and more recently, Richard Rorty and Stanley Fish (easy to read).[1] Revolutionary

1 I can understand neither the primary nor the secondary sources of Heidegger, so I've given up; despite the difficulty of Lacan and Derrida, there are good secondary sources; for example, the chapter on Lacan by Malcolm Bowie in John Sturrock's *Structuralism and Since* (Oxford: Oxford University Press, 1979), and the chapter on Derrida by Jonathan Culler in the same book. Wittgenstein is horrible to read but *How to Read Wittgenstein* (London: Granta Press, 2005) by Ray Monk is excellent; Rorty's *Contingency, Irony, and Solidarity* (Cambridge: Cambridge University Press, 1989) is a primary source and good reading, as is Fish's *There's No Such Thing as Free Speech: And It's a Good Thing, Too* (New York: Oxford University Press, 1994).

thinkers, Nietzsche and Freud were standard-bearers for the modern and postmodern world. Those who talk this way are also called deconstructionists or, by those who want to insult them, relativists. Since there are many versions of truth, no interpretive community has a final say, although each person believes in the system he's adopted.

The psychiatrists and philosophers who operate deconstructively would like to think that they need no system, that their modern or postmodern system is self-immolating. At the same time, those accused of being relativists or nihilists don't want to be thought of as asses, advocates of "anything goes." They exonerate themselves from the charge of relativism by having a high interest in argument and debate, not because argument will lead to the right answer, but because argument can discredit cultures that mistreat women, are fascistic or colonial, and in psychiatry, reveal the silliness of things like curing patients through love—the tactic of Marilyn Monroe's psychiatrist, whose methods I'll discuss in the following chapter.

I'm cheering for the psychiatrist who approaches her patient *post*scriptively rather than *pre*scriptively; that is to say, she studies what he does or has done—never what he ought to do in the future. She neither explicitly identifies nor preaches on behalf of her deconstructive methods, nor does she explain how they work or why they matter. She gets the idea across with her attitude, her style, her way of talking, with the result that most patients become interested in this unexpected style of detective work.

To completely avoid platitudes is impossible, yet the psychiatrist attempts to do just that. Many psychiatrists are better than I am at coming up with nonstandard interpolations—humorous, ominous, weird—commentaries that remind me of postmodern novels and strange abstract art. Such postmodern deconstructive talk pressures the patient to consider new ways of thinking. For example, Nabokov's novel *Pale Fire*, much admired by those who know about such things, left me cold. Were it assigned to me as a test or as homework, I could figure out the novel—I was always a conscientious schoolboy—but for simple pleasure I'm too lazy. But it's pertinent to the subject of change. That I have such a limitation is not as much of a problem as I sometimes think because what I'm good at is my psychological *attitude*, listening relentlessly and endlessly puzzling over what my patient says, an attitude radically different from day-to-day conversational style. Jacques Derrida and Jonathan Winters have remarkable off-the-wall verbal skills; I aim to be a cautious Oscar Wilde or a quiet Robin Williams, but what I'm best at is avoiding have-a-nice-day talk.

I call such talk nonstandard discourse—exaggeration, unusual angles on things, even resorting to the bizarre. To Robin Williams and other comedians, such talk comes naturally; for me, it's hard work. I was reminded of this recently when I was in the Museo Nacional de Antropología here in Mexico City. A tag on an exhibit reported that in the eleventh century, the Chichimec tribe arrived from the north of Mexico. Led by Mixcóatl, one of the bands settled in Culhuacán. While hunting, Mixcóatl came across a woman named Chimálmatl. As she stood naked, Mixcóatl shot four arrows without harming her. This happened again until finally he caught and possessed her. From this union was born Quetzalcóatl, the god most commonly heard about in Mexico. It fascinates me that the central god of the Mayans had been conceived in the drama of rape. This is the kind of story I like to latch onto in order to stir things up with my patient, a story that isn't "nice" and that makes him think. Although most of the time we don't pay much attention to such stories, there's actually a long tradition about new beginnings, both in history and in mythology, of sacrificing something wonderful to the gods: virgins, unblemished animals, first drops of wine. Other rapes in mythology include Zeus's rape of Europa and the founding of Europe, the rape of the Sabine women and the founding of Rome, Hades' rape of Proserpine and the creation of the seasons, Paris's rape of Helen that sparked the Trojan War.

Strangely, these rapes are two-faced, savagery and ecstasy snapped together; even stranger, the words rape and rapture have a common etymology. Such myths change our thinking—evil becomes good, realities shift—and since helping people to change is the psychiatrist's job, a psychiatrist has to take these myths seriously.

Here is an example in which I behave in a way that violates the standard rules of how a psychiatrist should conduct an initial interview. There's not much in the way of brilliant thinking, nor are my metaphors as dramatic as the myth of Mixcóatl, but my talk is unexpected enough to stir things up, the thing that leads to change. My reflections? The goings-on during the appointment are pretty insane except it's *me* who is strange, with eccentricities tolerable only because of the grim (earnest? quizzical? insistent?) seriousness with which I say unexpected things.

It's November 2011, and Anneliese Muther has phoned to book some time with me. During our appointment, Mrs. Muther will have a hand in how I talk to her, and I will have a hand in how she talks to me. As Montaigne said, "When I'm playing with my cat, how do I know she's not playing with me?" Although she and her family have a cottage near mine, I've never met Mrs. Muther. She is German but has lived in Canada for many years.

Meeting #1

"Could I see your insurance card?" I say. I read her name: Anneliese Henderson Muther. "Henderson?" I say, as I write down her information.

"My mother is proper. She's German, but she liked the Englishness of the name Henderson."

"So have you turned into a proper English lady?" A silence. I notice she's handsome and healthy looking, flashing her black eyes. *Is her blouse too tight, a bit dishevelled? Low class?* I also notice she's tall and nicely rounded with a bit of plumpness she carries well.

"That's the problem. I'm not proper. My mother is a good person, but my father is awful, drinks too much, bosses everyone around. I'm lucky because Tommy—he's my husband—is a nice guy."

"You're not proper?"

"I'm having an affair with an older man." She looks me in the eye.

"I see," I say. "I guess you're awful like your father?" Her eyes widen just for an instant. She's alert, leaning forward a bit, wondering about the tricky turn this conversation is taking.

Then she giggles. "I've been in jail too. A friend of mine and I got caught with marijuana in Florida and spent a night in jail."

"And Tommy? I guess he's sweet and nice like your mother? Doesn't mind if you have an affair?"

"He doesn't know about it. What do you mean? I haven't told him, if that's what you mean." She pauses, obviously thinking about something, and watches me warily. "Well, that's part of it. I go out in the evening and he doesn't ask any questions. I even went to Montreal with Dan—he's my lover—and my husband just went along with me when I said I'd be gone for the night. Dan swept me off my feet. He is sort of different, quietly sure of himself, not a typical alpha male, but I guess that's what he is. He's an executive in our company, pretty important guy. We women in the office used to make jokes about a lot of the men in the office, how ridiculous it would be to have an affair with them, how incompetent they'd turn out to be, but we didn't make jokes about Dan. With Dan, I finally knew what sex could be like, that it was connected with love. It's not that my body didn't work before—I had orgasms and everything—but with this man it's very different. He wants me to leave Tommy so we can be together—and I'm thinking about it."

"Do men like you?" I say.

Carefully, she says, "Well, I suppose so..."

I take a chance, a risky speculation. "Do women like your father?"

"What do you mean?" I can see she is annoyed. "I'm not sure about the way you ask questions. A bit discourteous, don't you think?"

The word *discourteous* catches my attention, and I realize she is well spoken, uses language properly, has good diction. "You used the word *discourteous* just now," I say. "Is that word a bit formal, not so common in everyday speech? You must be interested in words, and if so, where did you get that interest? Does anyone else in your family like words—your mother, perhaps, who liked the name Henderson?"

She looks at me with narrowed eyes, then seems suddenly to realize that I'm doing detective work, and that she might join in. "No, it's my father, not my mother. He went to university, but he's a boor. He likes literature, even poetry. I'm like him in that regard."

Again, I notice: *in that regard*.

"Our time is up," I say. "Can you come at this time next week?"

She brushes against me as she leaves the office.

I've asked neither why she's come nor about symptoms—I've attended only to what was in front of my eyes. But in that short time, I've stirred things up a bit, which might lead to Mrs. Muther viewing herself differently.

THERE ARE OTHER kinds of change, the most important of which is how powerfully we humans respond to suggestion: hypnosis, the placebo effect, canned laughter, propaganda, advertising, pep talks, inspirational sermons, ominous background music. But in the psychiatric business things are never simple; a person who follows a suggestion may not have changed at all, may simply be acting in character, conforming in his typical style. I have to admit my suspicion that most of the good results of psychiatric treatments are due to suggestion, including the favourable outcomes both of psychotherapies and of medications. If I tell someone who has been treated with antidepressant medication that about 70 percent of people have a good result from taking that drug, then add that roughly the same percentage of patients given sugar pills also have a good result, I earn an enemy for life. (Seventy percent is an old figure. My students tell me that these days the improvement rate is less. This puzzles me because the results of most psychiatric treatments have always hovered around the 70 percent figure. This excludes the subgroup of patients said to have schizophrenia, who of course can't tell us they are better because they've not thought of themselves as unwell in the first place.) If I tell a one-time psychotherapy patient that the psychotherapy cure resembles being cured like a ham—it's actually an apt metaphor—I might be murdered.

Those given antidepressants (or sugar pills) use words like *cured* and *improved*; those who have talking doctors use the word *helped*. Despite the pallid word *helped*, those who see talking doctors are satisfied, if not smug. Although they rarely say they've been cured, they do say they've changed for the better, a change they believe to be profound, more sophisticated and thorough than that experienced by those who've merely swallowed a pill—propaganda learned from me and other talking doctors. Don't misunderstand; when I trained to be a psychoanalyst many years ago, I was myself in psychoanalysis, learning a way of thinking I'm glad I didn't miss. But that's an opinion, therefore as brittle as porcelain. Obviously, like any other experience, it changed me, but it's moot whether I'm healthier, cured, or healed. When I was in training, almost all my fellow students were also in analysis and, even then, we wondered whether we had actually changed because of our psychoanalytic experience. But we made jokes: "Sadder but wiser"; "Wiser but poorer"; "Well, I now ask for correct change when overcharged twenty cents." Yes, out of the mouths of impoverished students and humourists when paying $800 (in 2016 dollars) for seeing one's analyst five times a week. Don't misunderstand; I'm glad I did it, and if there's a lingering rancour, I'm not aware of it.

A hundred years ago, before the current explosion of modern mythological psychiatric diseases, and before visiting a psychiatrist became a commonplace, a similar percentage of troubled people, having received the then-current psychiatric "treatments," would have reported that they were better. Like all psychiatrists, and because they reflect well on me, I like reports of improvement in my patients. We doctors are forever impressed by what happens in our offices—and we should know better.

Human change is as elusive as quantum physics. Both the physicist's and the psychiatrist's acts of observation mess things up because the presence of an observer affects the data being studied. When the psychiatrist gathers evidence, she finds herself so involved that she becomes part of what's going on, a shareholder in what she's listening to and studying. That's the nature of the treatment—to investigate a life so carefully that in an unexpected way the psychiatrist becomes part of what has to be studied. Most of all, the psychiatrist helps her patient to loosen his stereotyped ways, to become more imaginative. Reining in her own ordinariness, she comes up with novel ideas about what she herself does and about what she hears from her patient.

Whatever change the patient achieves has little to do with happiness—although patients often *say* they are happier. Happiness and unhappiness are part of life, and the psychiatrist can't do more than give her patient a nudge in a direction that he decided to pursue by consulting her—to rethink things and act less stupidly. Happiness is not part of the contract. Changing is a struggle, wrestling with a predecessor or an archetype. To become Marilyn Monroe, Norma Jean Baker had to compete against the iconic women of history like Lola Montez, Salomé, Theda Bara; to write this book, I had to compete with iconic psychiatrists: Emil Kraepelin, Sigmund Freud, and my teacher, Karl Menninger. These attempts changed me. The goal is not perfection and might not even be improvement; rather, it is to make a shift, re-examine some self-damaging habits, *attempt* to rethink who one is, to rewrite one's biography. Whoever re-examines things sees the world differently, the universe in which he lives is changed forever, even if his surface foibles, choices, habits, and interests look the same.

The patient brings to his appointments his preferred stories—what else could he bring? By focusing on stories, teasing them apart, and finding parallels, contradictions, and purposes in them, the patient and psychiatrist together open up new vistas, a new language, and new metaphors for what's going on. If he becomes interested, the patient will learn something, devise new interpretations of who he is. Diluted by new dramas, his previous worries, preoccupations, and ways of living will be put in perspective, sometimes vanish. But the psychiatrist can't prove this, and her self-doubt is crucial; it allows for even more stories, revisions, analogies, and paradoxes. Without doubt of her own positions, the psychiatrist can't entertain new ones. So when she's unsure—I mean this to be distinct from dithering—that uncertainty is a strength, one her patient will identify with.

If the patient shows little interest in the work, the psychiatrist has to wake him up; the responsibility for the treatment is hers. I sometimes hear that a patient is unsuitable, is not psychologically minded, isn't motivated—insulting and moralistic statements. I say to such a psychiatrist, "Get off your ass. In the operating room, the patient doesn't do the surgery." The patient doesn't visit a doctor frivolously; his life is at stake in such conversations. So if the patient isn't interested in what's going on, trot out that surgical model: it's analogous to a bleeding artery in the operating room, time for the psychiatrist to move into action. Any change that happens is a consequence of the psychiatrist's attitude, a peculiar and intense determination to figure out why her patient isn't interested in his own well-being. Instead of urging, persuading, explaining, and other pep-talk nonsense, the psychiatrist is persistently experimental, playful, poetic, amused, puzzled-out-loud and, oozing mildness, fiddles with, ponders, and attacks her patient's lack of interest in why he is running his life aground.

ALL THIS IS complicated by psychiatry at large. Psychiatric treatment is a ramshackle affair; psychiatrists are divided into tribes with different opinions on how patients are to be helped. Biological psychiatrists interpret their patients' words as referring to some type of abnormal biology, which they most commonly treat with drugs. These psychiatrists have little interest in highfalutin things like interpretive communities, deconstruction, and tribal identifications. But I have to be careful about scoffing because drugs do change people. Most create physiological changes that calm people down, and like any other event, the act of giving of pills will have its own effect, will change some people psychologically. As a short-term treatment, most drugs do little harm, but held to be a specific treatment for a disease, the administration of drugs invites trouble, invites patients to think of themselves as victims and no longer agents of their own ways of life. Yet despite my concerns, a pill can lead to both bad and good psychological effects. Anything—a wink, going bald, being prescribed a pill by a kind doctor—can lead to a change for the better or the worse.

Empty theoretical pronouncements are everywhere in the psychiatric literature, apparent in a review published in the *Canadian Medical Association Journal*, a respected and refereed publication.[2] Despite its large, full-colour illustrations of a brain and a brain synapse, the article is immediately invalidated by its frequent use of phrases such as "are likely," "suggests that," or "it is possible that," statements that aren't scientific. What follows is the official précis of the article that, in the journal, appears in a bulleted list placed in a call-out box at the beginning. Keep in mind that this is a prestigious journal, its articles screened by anonymous referees and so-called experts who should have used their expertise to dismiss the article as the trash that it is. The summary is such a long list of unwarranted assumptions that I'm unsure where to start. I have underlined the deadly, self-undermining phrases, and in square brackets, I've interleaved my own comments:

> Major depressive disorder is caused by the cumulative impact of genetics, adverse events in childhood and ongoing or recent stress. [*This statement contains no information. Everything about me, including my cultural interests, the texture of my skin, and the way my liver*

---

2 M. aan het Rot, S.J. Mathew, and D. Charney, "Neurobiological Mechanisms in Major Depressive Disorder," *Canadian Medical Association Journal* 180, no. 3 (Feb. 3, 2009): 305–13.

metabolizes glycogen, is also caused by the "cumulative impact of genetics, adverse events in childhood and ongoing or recent stress." It is an empty "people breathe" or "people speak a language" statement. Everything about me is caused by the "cumulative impact" of plenty of things in addition to genes, adverse events, and stress. For example, the culture I live in, the food I've eaten during my lifetime, the inspiring people I've worked with, the books I've read, and my private successes and joys.]

Gene-environment interactions seem to predict a person's risk for major depressive disorder better than genes or environment alone. [*Another empty claim—explicitly confessed by the authors' phrase "seem to." Once again, the sentence contains no information and has nothing to do with science. It would help if these people would tell me something about human beings that is* not *a product of gene-environment interaction.*]

Structural and functional brain abnormalities in patients with major depressive disorder may be associated with low levels of brain-derived neurotrophic factor, abnormal function of brain-derived neurotrophic factor, abnormal function of the hypothalamic-pituitary adrenal axis and glutamate-mediated toxicity. [*Impressive-sounding words, all cancelled by admitting that major depressive disorder "may be associated with" something or other. Structural and functional brain abnormalities may be associated with my sexual preferences and my tooth-brushing habits, for example, even though in neither depressives nor in me can such things be demonstrated.*]

These abnormalities are thought to contribute to recurrent episodes of major depressive disorder and chronic illness. [*Not "thought to" by me, so what does this statement prove? Opinion proves nothing: some people are of the opinion that astrology explains depression better than science.*]

Existing options for antidepressant treatment are limited by their delayed onset of action, lack of efficacy and adverse outcomes. [*Of course there is a delay before patients get better. We psychiatrists have always known that, although it's not immediate, depressed people usually recover spontaneously. As distinct from schizophrenia, which follows a chronic downhill course, major depression is defined by the fact that these patients have spontaneous remissions. That's one of the reasons why studies of the effectiveness of antidepressants are useless.*]

> Future developments include the advancement of personalized medicine by means of genotyping for interindividual variability in drug action and metabolism. [*This is good public relations, but what has it to do with scientific medicine?*[3] *And as for genotyping, hopes for the predictive powers of the much-vaunted human genome project are fading fast.*[4]]

If you argue with a psychiatrist, you're liable to break your shins, so prepare in advance, then hold her feet to the fire. Ask these questions: "Is there any known biological cause that occurs in every case of depression (or any other psychiatric disorder, including schizophrenia)? Can you diagnose depression using *any* biological evidence or test? Am I right that the diagnosis of depression is made by talking to the patient, by studying his social behaviour?"

Despite my debunking of psychiatric myths and my strong arguments in favour of taking apart the patient's established world of memories, opinions, and actions, have I gotten anywhere? The best answer is probably "perhaps." After many months of doing analytic psychotherapy with a patient, it may just have been an intellectual exercise. A close look at the patient once he is done shows that cynics are still cynics, Roman Catholics are still Roman Catholics, and fans of the bullfight are still fans of the bullfight. Freud hoped that a good analysis would dissolve belief systems (in a paper called "The Future of an Illusion" he argued that a psychoanalytic treatment was incomplete if the patient was still religious), but the truth is that the treatment ends with the fundaments of the patient's character intact. Perhaps we can say that, like most human events, intensive psychotherapy changes us but does not transform us.

I WRITE BOOKS because I want to improve the way psychiatry is practised—at least that's the story I've told myself until this very moment, this minute when I'm looking for an example of how rewriting a story changes the writer's life. How can I change, in other words? Can I

---

3 D.B. Goldstein, "Common Genetic Variation and Human Traits," *New England Journal of Medicine* 360, no. 17 (April 23, 2009): 1696–8.

4 Roger Collier, "Popping the Genetics Bubble," *Canadian Medical Association Journal* 184, no. 6 (April 3, 2012): 637–8.

rewrite the story I've told myself all these years? The new story will be one I've not thought of before, something less self-serving than "I write books in order to improve psychiatric practice." You don't know me, but I do, and I know that during several years of my childhood I was a discriminated-against outsider. So could it be that when I subvert the way psychiatry is currently practised, I'm having my revenge on the establishment, on the powers that be, the powers that once made me an outsider? In that new scenario, "I'll fix those establishment bastards" is the reason behind writing books. This doesn't mean my critique of psychiatry is wrong or that it's not true that I want to improve psychiatric practice; it just means that I've told myself a new story, one in which I'm not simply a book-writing hero as I thought ten minutes ago. Rewriting a personal narrative has just this dramatic effect: it changes us; we are no longer the person we were before. And if circumstances and intelligence come together as they should, our patients can change too.

Thus the cure the patient once hoped for becomes ambiguous. Among other things, he finds himself consoled by the weird realization that there *is* no consolation. It's worse: ever-present is the danger that a consolation—for example, the psychiatrist's important-sounding comments—looked at in the cold light of day will turn out to be tired clichés. The final insult is that when I talk about the nitty-gritty of the cure, try to steer you, the reader, toward the heart of the matter, it's only my confabulation of what's going on. What can be said absolutely about change and cure is disappointing, a whimper:

In every society, some troubled people visit a culturally recognized expert; those people and their gurus have unusual, emotionally laden dealings with one another; the dealings are conducted in a ritualized language—in Western culture, all too often in the language of disease and treatment or in the language of psychoanalysis and its derivatives.

In the words of Shakespeare, from *Henry IV*:

> [the] bringer of unwelcome news
> Hath but a losing office, and his tongue
> Sounds ever after as a sullen bell ... (1.1.100–102)

There is no clear statement to be made about change. Sometimes, it's peace of mind or new-found assertiveness; having been talked about, a beloved wife is transformed into a bore or a shrew, someone who ought to be divorced (am I then a marriage buster?). Or a ridiculous mother, her primitive emotionality maddening, comes to look different; her passions, because in the service of kindness, no longer seem histrionic. What the patient realizes is that rethinking things, the life of the mind, is both an enrichment of life and a consolation for the hurts of life.

This is all nonsense, of course, because I'm trying to "explain" something that can't be explained: change. So how does the treatment end? Well, maybe the patient becomes fed up, glad to be rid of the psychiatrist who has been stirring him up. Another patient, in a delirium of interest in his treatment, will leave reluctantly, broken-hearted to lose his doctor. In that case bereavement counselling will be necessary—everybody needs bereavement counselling, don't they? Or so the media tell me.

11

How to Stay Meta with Marilyn

We are what we pretend to be.

KURT VONNEGUT

IN 1953 I worked for the summer at the Banff Springs Hotel in Alberta. Because all of us who worked there were students, we had great fun. And there was a perk—that year, while making films in the Canadian Rocky Mountains, many Hollywood stars stayed at the hotel. We got to rub shoulders with Alan Ladd, Shelley Winters, Robert Mitchum, and best of all, Marilyn Monroe—all guests at the hotel for many weeks. We liked Marilyn Monroe best because she was modest. She didn't dress flamboyantly, flounce around, or wear makeup. Self-effacing, she came into the hotel using the garbage entrance because when she came in through the lobby there was too much commotion. Some of the other stars were vulgar, showing off in the lobby to be sure people knew they were there. When we did errands for her, Marilyn answered the door of her room herself, and gave decent but not extravagant tips. And there was a bonus: Joe DiMaggio came to visit her. Most of us saw her on location or saw what the newspapers reported, that she held things up by staying in her tent for no obvious reason. But we all loved her.

At the end of her stay, Ms. Monroe sent a notice to the staff saying she appreciated our help so much that she wanted to put on a show for us in our recreation hall, and so she did. Unfortunately for me, I had to work that night. But a few days later, when I punched the time clock, the bulletin board was filled with photos of Marilyn's performance. I didn't recognize the innocent young woman who'd spent the summer in the hotel. Over the course of the summer, I'd forgotten the red lips, the wild hair, the tight dresses, and the postures. It unsettled me. In the photographs of her show, she seemed to have transformed herself into another person. Through the years, I've often thought about that fabulous ability she had to metamorphose from one incarnation of womanliness to another, to hold within herself such contrasting social practices. But there is something else, something that everyone with eyes to see knows: Marilyn Monroe was a honeytrap.

Instead of saying she had a psychiatric illness, a disorder with a cause, I'm going to use a different language: I say Marilyn Monroe was a swindler. The idea is that when she thought of herself as a victim, someone afflicted with a disease, she wasn't doing herself a favour. If she had done the opposite, thought of herself as having a hand in her crazy behaviour, she might have had a better payoff. Had she been my patient, I'd have told her she was a swindler—but coaxingly, with a twinkle in my eye, hoping I could get her on my side in the attempt to shift her view of herself. Since all of us are swindlers, offering up unique personas that inevitably include our own version of talented craziness, my odd use of language doesn't demand a great imaginative shift. Ralph Greenson—Ms. Monroe's psychiatrist—should have done this, invited her to notice what she was up to, not necessarily using my "swindler" language, but by choosing any metaphor that contradicted the idea of victimhood. But he didn't. Greenson never helped her to see that, in her own way, she was as talented a swindler as the rest of us. He accepted at face value the archetypal images she showed him—she showed them to everyone—that as well as being a star, she was damaged goods, the passive victim of a mental flaw. The other archetypal image she enacted, the double-barrelled sexpot, both a provocative vamp and a needy, eyelash-fluttering innocent—he seemed to ignore.

If I'd had a chance, I would have told Greenson to "stay meta" (that pretentious but important word again), insisting that his aim when he spoke to Ms. Monroe should not have been to respond in kind when she defined herself as helpless and weak. Instead his aim should have been to make comments about her determination, her resolve, to define herself that way, to sell the world on the idea of her vulnerability. I would have insisted that he reclassify what she said, redefine her suggestions of personal weakness as being nothing more than ideas that served her purposes, purposes so far unknown. He ought never to have gone along with MM's intent; instead, he should have said only things like, "You seem to be setting up a situation in which I am supposed to see you as vulnerable and tragic." And to limit his own miscalculations of what was going on, he should have been asking the same type of question of himself: "What situation am I trying to set up here?" and, "To what extent am I buying into her story, the one that messes her up?"

The point is that no one knows anything about us but what we choose to display. What Ms. Monroe revealed was dramatic, made to order for moviegoers and the wider public, none of which had anything to do with illness or disease. Because she was a person, she *did* things, and this property of doing things is what her talking doctor should have been interested in. Ms. Monroe had goals and aims, and when he was with her, Greenson was her audience, so she would have performed according to her idea of what effect she wanted to have on him. Greenson would have also been theatrical, and just as actively as she did for him, he would have performed for Ms. Monroe—who was *his* audience. To recap: as opposed to lumpy objects, people are interactive and theatrical—as Shakespeare taught us in *As You Like It*.

> All the world's a stage,
> And all the men and women merely players;
> They have their exits and their entrances,
> And one man in his time plays many parts. (2.7.139–142)

Greenson assumed his patient was handicapped and was determined to play out the role of the intellectual Professor Higgins in *My Fair Lady* who saves the destitute flower girl, Eliza Doolittle. Obviously, had I been her psychiatrist, my first reaction would have been to think of her just as Ralph Greenson did—that she was a poor soul, childish and innocent. But Greenson didn't just notice that reaction; he *believed* in the Professor Higgins/Eliza Doolittle story he was living out with Ms. Monroe. He forgot the first thing a student psychiatrist is taught: "Don't take at face value what your patient tells you. Never write in your case report that 'The patient's mother neglected him.' Instead, write, 'The patient *reports* that his mother neglected him.'" Beware of taking the patient's precious words literally.

BEING A TALKING doctor is complicated because all of us have personal hang-ups, so things are always difficult, so difficult that our work has earned the title of "The Impossible Profession." One of the hard things to remember is that everything our patients do is a communication, that their actions tell us who they are or, more accurately, tell us about the image they want to project, their preferred identity. It's not play-acting, hokum, or fakery; it's vital, and it's done with energy and skill. Even a fool and a loser are passing on what to them is an essential message: "Take note of the fact that I am a fool; it's the image of me you're to keep in mind, and don't ever think of me as smart or competent." Or "I'm a loser, and I insist that's to be in the foreground of your mind—get it?" Through words, body language, facial expressions, hairstyle, and clothes, everyone communicates who he is determined to be, who he thinks he is, and who he wants us to think he is—including every psychiatric patient. It's not simple; behaviour is a cornucopia of symbols, clues, and cues, impossible to figure out except in bits and pieces. To make things worse, every affirmation includes its opposite: "If I seem sure of myself, I'm signalling that you are never to see me as insecure, but secretly, I'm also signalling that if you change the language you're using, you can say that I'm covering up, that I *am* insecure."

Since every patient presents himself as unwell, it's easy to forget that complaints are complicated and to immediately think repair is in order, neglecting to think about why the patient presents himself as he does. The complexity of human communications makes it necessary to react with concern, but also to think otherwise. Since the psychiatrist's job is to help, concern is automatic and not taking weakness and vulnerability at face value is hard. It's where Ralph Greenson, Marilyn Monroe's psychiatrist, fell down on the job.

While I was doing my training, Ralph Greenson published a book on psychoanalytic technique. The book was logical and filled with common sense. If this, he said, do that. And if that, do this. If you're five minutes late for an appointment, give the patient an extra five minutes at the end of the appointment, or an extra five minutes the next day. If the patient asks, "Why don't you answer questions?" explain that your chief interest is in his fantasy of why you don't answer questions. If the patient asks again or complains, stay silent. This made sense to me; for a young rationalist, the book had been sent from heaven. After reading Greenson, I thought I knew exactly what to do. But now I know better.

Of course talking doctors want to say the right thing, but it's also true that it's impossible to *pre*script what is to be said. Life—and the psychiatric setting is real life—is more complicated than that. What do you say if your best friend suggests that you should take his wife out to dinner, even though he saw her stroking your arm earlier? What if you want to tell off the professor who singled you out and mentioned your heaviness in front of the class, but who, in a few months, will assign you a mark that may be decisive for you to get into graduate school? What if your boss is touchy about criticism and is about to make a bad decision? These are thorny questions, which is why it's impossible to make a rule for what the psychiatrist ought to say.

Many reports can be found on the Internet about Greenson's therapeutic methods with Monroe in 1962. The best documented are those recorded in Lois Banner's biography, *Marilyn: The Passion and the Paradox*. Since Ms. Monroe had previously seen several famous psychoanalysts, and perhaps after he himself had tried doing analytic work with her, Greenson made a terrible decision. He assumed that, not only did Marilyn Monroe have a disease that needed to be treated, but her disease was so severe, so disabling, that she was incompetent, not well enough to profit from the talking cure, not as competent a person as you and me.

Greenson concluded that while Ms. Monroe's vamp behaviour was a skill set, the maiden-in-distress behaviour was *not* a skill set, and the latter was a direct manifestation of inner decrepitude. Having decided that this was a deficit, a debility, Greenson felt he had to stand in for certain missing functions, needed to treat her as a mental amputee who he needed to put on a life support system. Life would be impossible were we humans not kind to one another, but as a treatment, if it is presumed to be the essential curative ingredient, kindness is deadly, a kind of artificial friendship or parenting. A psychiatrist who gives medication to a patient who has no disease has the same anti-therapeutic effect, strongly conveying to her patient the idea that he is disabled. Some patients want this, ask for medications, but that a patient has a taste for such things is far less important than doing what's medically proper.

Greenson's theory must have gone like this. "This patient, Marilyn Monroe, is undeveloped and flawed (that is to say, she truly has an abnormal ego, a state analogous to having abnormal chemicals in the brain) and that's why she doesn't leave her tent and do her scenes. It's why she changes suddenly from helpless maiden to vamp; it's why she is promiscuous and has failed at three marriages. She has a defect in her judgment faculty and a defect in the faculty that regulates impulse control." (As I will explain in chapter 20, faculty theory is comically naïve.)

And she did indeed do stupid things. She fell in love with many men, seduced them, and seduced others she didn't love; the men—surprise, surprise—fell like bowling pins. A photographer for whom she modeled early in her career was impressed by her uncanny ability to pose and be photographed. When the shoot was done, Ms. Monroe said something stupid to him: "Do you want to go in?" According to my (private) source, the photographer declined—to his later regret. "What a bragging point that would have been," he added. Greenson's idea must have been that the weak, helpless Marilyn Monroe was a real and diseased Marilyn, and that her dramatic femininity had only one function, to satisfy primitive, oral-dependent cravings (horrible jargon), a raw need to have people love and affirm her. I'm inclined to think she felt her femininity was her great power—and her great tragedy.

My guess is that, among other things, Greenson must have thought something like this: *Ms. Monroe is not a siren. Really, she is undeveloped, one of those innocent, sweet, and pure girls with creamy skin and delicate underwear.* In thinking this, he would have been in a state of belief about the archetype she was portraying, apparently forgetting that reality is iffy at the best of times and, in the case of human behaviour, always a way of presenting oneself to the world rather than a raw fact. I remind you that I briefly did the same thing when I received Wilma Chan's letter (chapter 7). Both Greenson and I assumed that our patients, Mrs. Chan and Ms. Monroe, were in a state of need rather than recognizing that they were both *presenting* themselves as needy, that they were waiting for us, the two rescuing Romeos, to awaken them, guide them into adult health. Like all of us, Greenson was powerfully influenced by his own naïveté, hoping upon hope that Marilyn Monroe was really a lonely Bangkok bargirl in disguise, waiting to be saved. *I only think of her as a patient or as a daughter*, he would have thought. *I'm the one who can save her*. The fantasy could, of course, just as easily have been another salvation—a cure by drugs, being reborn in Christ, or purification through a disciplinary strap, whip, or scolding.

We don't know how Marilyn spoke of herself, whether she used the language of disease when she spoke to her psychiatrist. But we do know that Greenson used that language. Most patients arrive in my office speaking of disease—it's their admission ticket—but within minutes, few still speak that language. By choosing to speak about their way of life rather than about disease, I steer them in a new direction, an alternative conception of themselves. It's not that I insist on talking about their way of life; a few simple questions get things going. Only a few go back to the disease story, either in that initial interview or in later appointments.

Somewhere within herself Marilyn Monroe would have realized that she'd triumphed beyond anyone's wildest dreams, had achieved a miracle in which she was loved and admired by millions, and now she'd triumphed with her psychiatrist as well, convinced him that she was a helpless waif. Such a situation has consequences of guilt, the same guilt suffered by countless other performers who have been wildly successful, only to kill themselves or sabotage their lives. Examples are Elvis Presley, Michael Jackson, Whitney Houston, Amy Winehouse, Robin Williams, and Philip Seymour Hoffman (it's interesting that successful athletes don't seem to commit suicide nearly as often).

As a psychoanalyst, Greenson should have recognized a familiar idea—that the last thing depressed people need is more love and attention. As a student psychiatrist, I was given a handout describing that the attitude taken toward depressed, suicidal patients should be "firm kindness." Not explicit in the handout was a modification explained only in words by my teachers. The kindness element had been withdrawn, replaced with "be firm and matter-of-fact." Prescribing attitudes for psychiatrists— in other words, asking them to fake it—is silly, but the awareness that out of guilt both depressed and celebrated people react badly to mushy and loving attitudes is worth keeping in mind.

Wild young girls from Helicon were trained by Apollo to be Muses, women who, through art and love, had the power to possess men's minds. As an expert in possessing men's minds, influencing her psychiatrist was a cinch for Marilyn Monroe. Why else would he have blundered so badly that, according to Banner's book, he took her to live in his home? Greenson's rationalization was that she needed, for the first time, to have the experience of a normal home and a concerned father. These nurturing strategies strike me as silly, conventional, pedestrian—and false.

At times, Greenson saw Monroe twice a day, and it is reported that on the day before she died he spent six hours with her. He even intervened in her business affairs. At one point, John Huston asked Marilyn Monroe to play the role of Anna O. (Josef Breuer's famous patient) in a film about Freud, but because of the objections of Anna Freud, the film was never made. Some time before, Ms. Monroe had seen Anna Freud professionally, but because professional confidentiality and neutrality are absolute, Ms. Freud should never, ever have interfered with what Monroe was up to; what MM did in her life was none of her analyst's business and, in addition, implies that MM was too stupid to decide for herself what to do, not a citizen worthy of full respect. Unfortunately, Greenson also blabbed about his famous patient. Greenson helped to kill the film about Anna O., professional neutrality and confidentiality be damned. And when Ms. Monroe missed many days of work on the never-completed film *Something's Got to Give*, 20th Century Fox was about to fire her, so Greenson personally guaranteed that she would come to the set and perform. His guarantee failed, and she was fired.

Moreover, Greenson arranged for Monroe to have a housekeeper, who reported to him about his patient's behaviour. On the night of Monroe's death, the housekeeper phoned Greenson at three in the morning. He came to the house, broke Marilyn Monroe's bedroom window (she had locked the bedroom door), and found her dead, her body stiffened by rigor mortis. Other reports say that Greenson was called at 10:00 p.m., that Bobby Kennedy was involved, and that there was a cover-up. For those interested, typing "Greenson Marilyn Monroe" into a Google search will yield a flood of articles about the details or imaginings of what happened.

Marilyn Monroe's maiden-in-distress presentation of herself isn't unique or unusual: it's an archetypal theme in Western culture and in all cultures. Our favourite fairy tales turn on it: Cinderella, Snow White, Sleeping Beauty. Nor is Marilyn Monroe's portrayal of herself as the world's most magnificent vamp unique or unusual. It too is an archetypal theme in our culture, in all cultures: Mata Hari, Josephine Baker, Eva Perón, Thetis-of-the-shining-breasts (Achilles's mother, loved by Zeus).

Here is what I want to say to Greenson:

> Get cracking, man. This rescue thing you're doing is very standard, a platitude, saving the maiden in distress. Don't you remember what they taught us during our training? Your job is to listen with the third ear, to not take your patient's words literally, to stay meta, to show her you won't let yourself settle into standard thinking—to rape your own mind, shake yourself up, devise new readings of what she is saying to you. This will set an example, teach her that she can also unsettle her own mind, understand what she's doing in new ways. But you're letting the opposite happen, letting her team up with you to hang onto a destructive cliché.
>
> Tell her, for example, something she knows already but that you and she are pretending not to notice, that she is so skilled at her way of life that even you, an old hand at the psychiatric game, are powerfully affected, in thrall to her, her doting caretaker, perhaps romantically enslaved as well. Although it's true that you are, in a way, her slave, Ms. Monroe will also see that you aren't surrendering to that, that you keep digging, poking, pushing, and, in a sense, raping her usual ways of thinking. Concerned, yes. Mollycoddling, definitely not. Point out that she is stubborn, determined to live out her old stories, and by your actions show her that although you'll watch, you are determined to stand for new ways of thinking, ones she's never thought of before—hell's bells, ways *you* haven't thought of before—honest almost to the

point of being harsh. Not that she has to act differently—it's that business about us not having the right to tell people to live their lives in any way other than they already do—but only that you will work with her to study everything she does.

But be careful. Don't take my rape metaphor too literally. We psychiatrists have tried many crude "rape" experiments already. Do you remember? Electric shocks, insulin shocks, lobotomies, ice-cold baths, isolation rooms? The rape I'm after is mostly about you, reinventing yourself and how you think about your patient. Never let up on the project of waking your own mind so you can make novel comments about what Ms. Monroe is up to. That our patients portray themselves in certain ways is one of the most important things we psychiatrists have to keep in mind. To use a nastier word—which you may get away with using if you do it tactfully—your bombshell patient is *masquerading* as a dependent baby, even living with Lee and Paula Strasberg (Monroe's drama coaches, creators of the school of method acting). They have taken her baby style literally, just as you do. She did it with her husband Arthur Miller too, always calling him "Papa," even before they were married.

Don't forget, Greenson, that she's been an accomplished siren for many years. I even imagine that she was a Shirley Temple when she was little, that all her life people responded to her with amazement, admiringly, enviously, resentfully. From the beginning she has had power, tremendous power—and still does. It's scary to be the most powerful woman in the universe, a reincarnation of Helen of Troy, who was also the most powerful woman in her universe; both Marilyn and Helen changed the world. We psychiatrists know that some people convince themselves that they can neutralize that terror by saying, "I'm weak, I'm helpless, I'm childlike, please take care of me." But cripes, surely we psychiatrists don't fall into the trap of believing such enactments, and reacting exactly like everyone else?

Alas, because he'd signed on to the cure by love and reparenting, Greenson wouldn't have paid attention. Chastised or not, he would have believed he *had* to work heroically to save Marilyn Monroe, a transference/countertransference problem run amok. Greenson was determined he would cure Marilyn Monroe of being Marilyn Monroe, a crazy misplaced hope. To say she was crazy is to say little, because, in one way or another, every one of us is crazy. The questions that count are always these: "What is Marilyn Monroe's way of being crazy?" "What is your way of being crazy?" "What is my way of being crazy?" (This book has plenty of clues.) "What is the girl next door's way of being crazy?"

> All the world's mad except for thee and me / And even thee's a little cracked.
> ANONYMOUS

If Ralph Greenson wasn't a little bit in love with Ms. Monroe, I'll eat my hat. What man wouldn't have been? But love doesn't mean courtship; it only means that talking doctors are human. I'm sure Marilyn Monroe was thrilled that she could seduce any man she chose, but she would also have had another hope: that she could *not* seduce any man she chose, especially her psychiatrist, from whom she needed something different. But sadly, she did seduce him—into seeing her as a baby—which was her duty, her destiny, and her nirvana. But it shouldn't have been Greenson's nirvana—he had a job to do.

Some women, especially handsome women, ask their psychiatrist about this explicitly. Marilyn Monroe would have had the question in mind: "How do I know that you're not going to get involved with me?" I've heard psychiatrists speak of how they respond when this question is posed, and I suspect Ralph Greenson would have given an answer similar to what I've heard others give: "No such thing can happen, Ms. Monroe," he would have said. "There will be no crossing of professional boundaries in this office, you can be sure of that."

Well, that answer makes sense. It's the way sensible people talk. But I don't like that answer, mostly because it isn't the truth. Here's the truth: "Life is unpredictable, Ms. Monroe, and that's what your question is about. You're hoping that even though you're the goddess of love, that even if we fall in love or I am an exploitative seducer, that I can foresee and guarantee something that can't be foreseen and can't be guaranteed."

MARILYN MONROE and Joe DiMaggio were checked out of the Banff Springs Hotel late in the summer of 1953 by my friend Don and another bellboy. Although I don't remember why, I was also on the elevator. Ms. Monroe, in a baby voice—a marvellously seductive baby voice—said to DiMaggio, "Don took care of me while you were away, Joe" (he'd been away on a business trip). It was a joke, but it was also her charm, her reference to her self-portrayal as the maiden in distress. She understood what she was up to better than her psychiatrist.

As you can see, I have plenty of advice for Ralph Greenson, but have I gotten to the bottom of things, figured out what makes psychiatry tick?

12

Storm the Citadel—or Melt It?

Prohibitions, cruel prohibitions, are what characterize a culture and make it work.
FRIEDRICH NIETZSCHE

WELL, YES. OF course the psychiatrist is storming the citadel. She is the mortal enemy of rigidities and miseries and stupidities long established. But she must also be careful; if she frightens the horses, nothing will have been gained.

In pre-Homeric times, Zeus enjoyed cruising the world, looking things over. Like many men, he had women in mind, especially young women, those still defending their sacred virginity. On the Asian side of the Bosporus, he spotted maidens playing on the beach, dancing, singing, skipping. Being girls, they weren't just having fun; they also had high hopes that if they were lucky a boy might come along. Like a wise psychiatrist, Zeus was careful not to frighten the girls, so he transformed himself into a beautiful white bull, walked across the beach, and lay down. Although they admired the bull's beauty, the girls were shy, and when he made deep lowing sounds, they giggled nervously. Eventually, they danced round him, patted his nose, and tied ribbons to his horns. One of them, Europa, climbed on his back. He stood up, walked into the sea, and swam away with Europa across the Hellespont all the way to Crete. There, he impregnated her and by doing so, founded Europe. In mythology, Europe isn't just there, its existence mysterious. It was *caused* by something—by a rape.

It's no coincidence that Zeus turned himself into a bull, then accomplished something both violent and mystical; the modern bullfight is a direct descendent of rapturous celebrations of bulls in ancient Crete. Matadors, asked about the bullfight, regularly refer to it as lovemaking—to Zeus making love to Europa—the most mutual and blissful of celebrations.

The ancient Greeks were smart, so they undermined the idea of a simple cause by making the story of Zeus and Europa ambiguous: when they were raped, many of the Greek women referred to the event as their "nuptials." *The Rape of Europa*, Titian's famous painting, depicts Europa lying on her back between the bull's shoulders and looking up blissfully as she is carried over the sea. In the water are horrible monsters; in the sky is a happy Eros, the messenger of Aphrodite, the goddess of love. By reminding you, my reader, that Europa thought of her encounter with Zeus as her nuptials, and by not bewailing the fate of a raped woman, I'm playing with fire, but since the talking treatment isn't just innocent chatter, I have no choice.

The early heroes of ancient Greece were embodiments of the bad part of this story; they occupied themselves with violence and non-stop war, killing one another and killing monsters. Since they were an army, I assume that, like soldiers everywhere, they practised military rape. Eventually, the gods grew fed up with these noisy, vulgar warrior-heroes. How did the gods solve the problem? The answer is obvious: with another rape. Paris raped Helen and ignited the Trojan War. As the gods intended, all the bloody-minded, old-style heroes were killed in the war, their barbarity brought to an end. In the new and changed world, heroes were different; they became talkers and thinkers. Odysseus, the man of twists and turns, survived by his wits; instead of killing the Sphinx with a weapon, Oedipus talked to her. This, it is said, was the birth of civilization—the prototype of change.

The moral of the rape story is that change is difficult. The psychiatric patient has built for himself a way of life that is a house of cards, a set of convictions that damage his life. But because it implies that a breath or a tap can knock it down, a "house of cards" is the wrong metaphor. More accurately, the psychiatric patient has created a way of life that is a fortress, a citadel, and it's hard for him to relinquish what's taken a lifetime to construct. Even "rocking the boat" is too gentle a metaphor for change; the psychiatric business, from start to finish, is a struggle. (In the bullring, that's what the bull is called: *toro de lidia*—the "bull of struggle.") And when things look good, when the work is seemingly going forward well, the psychiatrist and her patient are nearly always kidding themselves. In fact, the psychiatric experiment is eternal, so when things become safe, cozy, and optimistic, it's a sign that something has gone amiss; the parties to the conversation are "playing it safe." Similarly, if the matador is a coward, instead of drawing the bull close to himself with his cape, he will make fake passes, flamboyant passes that look spectacular and fool the uninformed, passes in which the bull's horn comes nowhere near the matador's body. The bull, too, may play it safe, search out a *querencia*, an area to which the bull retreats for safety. If a psychiatrist comforts herself and her patient with a cliché, she is conceding and inviting her patient to concede; both make concessions, basking in a cocoon of mutual admiration or any other of a thousand self-deceiving games.

In order to change, a patient—or any other person—needs something to perform against; without an impediment or a perceived lack, he languishes, and the psychiatrist must step into the breach and serve as just such an impediment. She dabbles, meddles with opinions, forces and propels events—indeed, she *creates* events. The metaphoric way out of the dilemma of stagnation is rape, not the metaphor of diagnosing, treating, and curing a disease. "What the devil do you mean by rape?" people ask. I have many answers:

- "What I've got in mind is a shock treatment."
- "I don't mean it in the sense of hurting someone. It's disestablishing some idols, derailing the misleading dreams my patient is living by."
- "I'm determined to loosen up the imaginary, the delusion, the unconscious fantasy, the complex, the archetype, the symbolic, and any other structure that screws my patient up."

- "It's giving up on that boilerplate, those clichés, those pep talks, and instead, throwing cold water in my patient's face and counting on doing it so skilfully that the patient will be able to say, 'Thanks, I needed that.' I also know that I can't just be provocative or earnest; I've also got to be witty and imaginative, using as much charm and determination I can muster."

These answers are both wrong and right and liable to make me an ally of my enemies—those colleagues who've decided that we've got to get our patients to behave better, who see patients as problematic people who need to shape up. My better answers are about me, less focused on male pugnacity and more focused on self-overcoming. They also invite the patient to do something new, to give up on platitudes, *to take risks*. This means sabotaging my own mind, shaking myself up, hoping I'll smarten up and stop thinking I'm supposed to tackle some imaginary flaw, lesion, or bad habit in my patients. It also means that as I smarten up, I'll find interesting ways of being an impediment to my patient's unhappy actions, impediments that are subtle yet resolute.

I'm trying to be cheeky, take risks, jerk myself around by slapping my own face, demanding of myself that I quit thinking I'm supposed to be passive and kind all the time, quit living in a millennia-old tradition that only helps me, me, me, relieves *my* nervousness and eases *my* revulsion when I have to deal with troubled and crazy people.

As I do my work, I'm envious of Theodor Geisel—"Dr. Seuss." He's into mischief: outrageous demands to eat green eggs and ham; intense pressure for children to do mischief while their parents are away. He's trying to one-up me with his metaphors, analogies in competition with my rape and bullfight metaphors. The best I can do is say that I can be gloriously raped by a man's bravery, and demoralizingly raped by a woman's submissiveness—and vice versa: I can be gloriously raped by a woman's glance, and demoralizingly raped by a man's cowardice.

I'm reminding you that unexpected circumstances provoke stories into existence, that a contrary event changes a person's life. Inspired by the death of his lover Patroclus, Achilles leads the Greeks to victory over the Trojans; when kissed (raped?) by Prince Charming, Sleeping Beauty's life changes forever; expelled from the Garden of Eden, Adam and Eve become free but burdened with the guilt of sin.

I'm referring to a principle both Dostoevsky and Nietzsche pointed to, and Ivan Karamazov's devil said it clearly: for change to take place, the devil must disturb the peace of the world. In the end, it will turn out that the devil is me, and if not, he will turn out to be you.

A LIBERAL AND DEMOCRATIC attitude is a psychiatric absolute—and a lot of hooey. This assertion should be no surprise: every absolutism (language game, symbolic order, interpretive community, ideology) is internally inconsistent. A thousand thousand capitalists find socialism to be preposterous; a thousand thousand socialists find capitalism to be preposterous, yet both ideologies are supported by logic. Unfortunately for all of us (I really mean "fortunately"), logic and reason aren't the superb instruments we assume them to be. The advocates of the Israeli and the Palestinian points of view don't hold to them because of logic; rather, their preference is just that—a preference, a taste, an opinion. Because each person loves the symbolic order he lives by, each person denies the impossibility of his own preferred world view. To paraphrase Jacques Lacan: the Real is so unknowable, so contradictory, and so paradoxical that every attempt to settle on a symbolic order has to be internally inconsistent; struggle and confusion, I say, are the order of the day.

The liberal stance of the psychiatrist, although crucial, is also stupid. Why? Because the patient, however ambivalently, is coming in order to change, so as well as being a liberal, the psychiatrist has to be a contradicting force, one or another kind of violator. Because she lives in her own symbolic order, to a certain extent this is inevitable—the personal convictions (the personal language games) of the psychiatrist inevitably contradict those of her patient. But the psychiatrist is ambitious, not content with a passive diffusion of her attitudes and stances toward her patient, and although she doesn't demand change, she pushes and nudges and nags. But if the psychiatrist inspires her patient, she has to be careful; she is always at risk of indulging in the Messiah complex, trying to inspire her *own* agenda, becoming another Kenneth Euston—my English fellow student from chapter 9—an Elmer Gantry, or a Jim Jones.

The psychiatrist pushes by being persistent and shrewd or sometimes humorous or ironic. She doesn't bother with small talk, makes no excuses, nor does she offer apologies—pathetic attempts to smooth things over—partly because one of her most important strategies is to be quiet. The psychiatrist's quietness is a provocation—like ambiguity, quietness pressures her patient to think. It is also a challenge. It transforms confident avowals into uncertainties, throws doubt on compliments and on complaints, and renders dubious any comment by the patient that things are worse or better. Emily Dickinson's poems—marvellously—end too soon, and therefore make us think. If the patient says he is doing better, that he is no longer taken in when his wife tells lies, the psychiatrist may not respond in words, but by way of quietness she implies, "What else can be said about this? Why do you emphasize the topic of 'improvement' today?" And when she does speak, the psychiatrist may make vague references to myths, movies, and popular stories, a vagueness that, like quietness, provokes her patient to think. When the psychiatrist notices herself becoming rational or intellectual or talkative, she worries, suspecting she is becoming a moralist.

Yes, to do your psychiatric job, you have to rock the boat, even if I'm your patient and even if I don't like it. You must play with my world, become a magician, turn things inside out and back to front, get things sparkling and whirling and kaleidoscopic. When doing your job properly, you'll stubbornly refuse the fixed positions that I have designed for myself, the fixed positions that cripple me. Nor will you go along with the fixed conventions of the world at large, clichés that might encourage me to stay the same.

But... what if the patient doesn't want the psychiatrist to be a contradicting force, to storm the citadel?

13

Tangential Logic

... like a fool... I oppressed her with gloom.
Truly, the world ought to belong to the singers and dancers!
J.M. COETZEE, *Waiting for the Barbarians*

JUST FOR THE Christmas holidays, there's an outdoor skating rink in the Zócalo of Mexico City, a scene ripe for Canadian analogies. Since almost none know how to skate, people are staggering around the ice, falling, laughing, having the time of their lives. It's warm today, twenty-five degrees, so this is hilariously funny. They stop the fun every couple of hours and just like at home, out comes the Zamboni to resurface the ice. Why don't I have to stamp my feet to keep warm? Why don't my nose hairs freeze when I breathe in? Why doesn't the wind sting? I'm coming back tonight, when I expect boys and maybe girls to be playing hockey, because skating rinks are different after dark, especially in the long Canadian nights. My mind conjures memories of sticks, pucks, and sounds from the ice, all better at night. Skates swoosh and scrape the ice, the air is brisk, sticks slap, the puck hits the boards—*thump, whump, thump*—an echo that's heard only at night, exaggerated by the white silence of snow. Layers and layers of memories from years ago, intact, as raunchy as ever. But it's too warm, so I'm wasting these memories here in Mexico.

Just north of the Zócalo is the Huey Teocalli (*Templo Mayor* in Spanish), which, five hundred years ago, was the religious heart of

Tenochtitlán, the capital of the Aztec empire. Although covered over by the Spanish city built by Cortés, it has now been excavated and—no surprise to a psychiatrist—it's been discovered that the Teocalli was rebuilt six times, each new temple covering the previous one. Like my hockey memories, the older versions of the temple are intact, memories of the past, alive and well, waiting to be ignited into alertness, nostalgia, or horror. The site reminds me of Freud's thought experiment about Rome. Freud was a serious man, but at the same time he had a playful mind, able to use associative logic:

> Let us imagine that Rome is not a populated city, but a person's mind with a long, event-filled past, a structure from which nothing that has happened has been lost, and earlier times of life still exist in memory alongside what is happening in the present... Where the Palazzo Caffarelli now stands, and without the Palazzo Caffarelli being removed, the temple of Jupiter Capitolinus also stands; and not only as it now is and as the Romans saw it, but also in its earlier forms, when it was Etruscan, and ornamented with ceramic roof ornaments... Where the Pantheon is we still find it as Hadrian gave it to us, but on the same site, the original building put up by Agrippa; indeed, the same building site would also support the church of Santa Maria sopra Minerva and the ancient temple over which it was built. And if we change our view, we can call up any of these images, one image or another.[1]

Freud's thought experiment refers to one of the most important things the psychiatrist does. Let's assume you've taken on the job of being my shrink again. If you talk about both my distant and recent past, including my childhood experiences and family, you'll have in mind a landscape that includes the ice-skating rink in the Zócalo, my boyhood hockey history, what I've read about the ancient versions of the Teocalli, and what Freud said about historical Rome. It's all in me, alive and influential, waiting for a posse—you and me—to hunt it down.

---

1 Sigmund Freud, *Civilization and Its Discontents* (Vienna: Internationaler Psychoanalytischer Verlag Wien, 1930), p. 10. First published as *Das Unbehagen in der Kultur* (*The Uneasiness in Culture*). My translation.

You, my psychiatrist, will help me to sniff out traces of previous choices, habits, hurts, and joys, and link them together.

Your interpretations will be made in a certain spirit: resolute neutrality, implying neither that you have unearthed abnormality or pathology nor suggesting your interpretations will cure something. Your disinterest—a synonym for neutrality—could suggest idleness or neglect. But for you, my psychiatrist, I assume it means earnest attentiveness. Making interpretations—translating ideas into a new form, inventing evocative new metaphors—is inevitable because once your conversation with me gets going, you never deviate from your meta-psychological stance. You'll find analogies in my history, from literature, and from anywhere in the social world.

Although the meta stance is disinterested, it also means that you, my doctor, have a job and a focus, an ironic focus that includes trouble, rapture, and delight—with an equal emphasis on everything. The associations, links, and analogies that are being uncovered—no, *invented*—will have a flavour: "Look at that," you'll say. "The connection we've just made shows how pervasive this pattern is in your life, that this grand/vile/banal way of thinking, the thinking that leads you to do *a*, *b*, and *c*, is more widespread, more deeply rooted than we realized before we made this connection/link/interpretation." Does anyone think she can discover a scientific cause for my tearful reaction to the memory of skate blades swooshing and cutting into the ice? To pucks thumping and echoing in the dark Canadian night? Someone could put a name on it, invent a metaphor—that I am a nostalgic fool, a faker, a researcher—but nothing is explained by a name.

Usually, but not always, I will pay close attention; after all, you shrinks don't talk much so I relish the things you actually say. As you cruise through my mind, listening without purpose, I can sense you're waiting for a click or a two plus two to equal four. An echo of what I've talked about on other occasions will catch your attention, a parallel, a pattern, or a habit never before connected to what you have noticed today. Or, contrariwise, you'll think of the opposite of what I've said; if I mention my toughness several times you'll wonder if I've got vulnerability on my mind. Your interpretations will sometimes be devilishly ingenious, an example of your odd mind in action. But it's risky—first, because if you don't watch your step it will turn out you've uttered a platitude, and second, because you may think you're interpreting *the* meaning, a final meaning, rather than interpreting *another* meaning, unique only to the degree that you and I haven't thought about me that way before. My narrated truths can be interpreted in dozens (hundreds, millions, an infinity) of ways, and if you're smart and imaginative, you'll figure out some of them. *The* meaning (metaphor, connection), a real/definitive/true meaning, does not exist. And no analogy or idea that's dreamed up is a cause—even though some of you psychiatrists have the bad habit of thinking you're interpreting the "cause" of things.

I'VE RECENTLY BEEN thinking about Richard Strauss's strange opera, *Die Frau ohne Schatten* (*The Woman without a Shadow*), wondering why, when I saw it in New York ten years ago, I'd found it so thrilling. *Such a stupid story*, I thought. *The fat soprano spent three hours bellowing and having conniptions because she didn't have a shadow*. Since it's highbrow opera, and since I aim to be a highbrow, I've been trying to figure this out.

I was born with a shadow, and as a child I loved it. It was a nuisance, too, because it was attached to my feet and I couldn't get rid of it. Sometimes I'd jump in the air, and just for a moment, I'd be free. Although in bright sunshine it obeyed the laws of nature, laws that weren't mine, at other times I could make my shadow obey *my* rules. I could, for example, walk toward a wall and make my shadow crawl up the wall and at the same time make it bigger. When I stood between streetlights, I had *two* shadows. My friends and I stomped on one another's shadows in some game I don't remember.

But there is a tragic end to this story. I no longer have a shadow—it has vanished. Although once central in my life, I haven't noticed my shadow for years. I have an apartment, a Rolex watch, a family, and a psychiatrist—you—but it's been decades since I've had a shadow. In *Die Frau ohne Schatten*, the dyer's wife is offered jewels and handsome men in return for her shadow, and that's what I've done—sold my shadow for material things. But this morning, after thinking about that tricky, beloved shadow of mine, I walked in bright sunshine past the wall of a condominium building site, and magically, there was my shadow again, as sprightly as ever, bopping along the hoardings beside me. Thinking about it brought my shadow back to life.

Similar tricks can be performed with a mirror. Because they reproduce movements too accurately, playing magic tricks with a mirror is only mildly interesting. It's nice to have a *Doppelgänger*, but that's about it. It's better looking into the distorting mirrors in a funhouse because there, the mirrors have something to say about how my twin in the mirror will act, as magical and thrilling as a magician, who also plays and fiddles with reality and with the world.

These are the secrets of your psychiatry business, but they also have something to do with art. The artist picks a scene, an image, or an idea, and plays with it—ironically, seriously, or with a sense of life's absurdity—just as I played with my shadow and my body and you play with my words. But with art, other things are in play: talent, taste, fashion, beauty—even advertising. Such parallels and analogies are the common stuff of all shadow play, including the childlike shadow play that goes on here in your psychiatric office. Not simply duplications or repetitions, analogies are themes, things I'm inventing, brilliant errors and evocative mismatches, resemblances that prepare me for action. Opposites are parallels denied. It seems, Doc, that in your psychiatric system:

- "My mother let me down after my brother was born" is a parallel to "When my wife has a baby, she will let me down."
- "My father was a brilliantly intellectual socialist but couldn't provide for our family" is both a parallel to and the opposite of "I'll become a lawyer-socialist with powerful, well-financed, trade-union connections."
- "I'm never feminine and sexy because if I were, I'd end up giving blow jobs to men the way our neighbour gave a blow job to my father."
- "I vehemently admire my husband, think of him as my hero because if I didn't, I'd overpower him, turn him into a wimp the way my mother turned my father into a wimp."
- "I'm independent and tough because were I to yield, I'd be a sissy like all the other men in my family."

If you draw my attention to a parallel I haven't thought of before, it's a surprise; if it contradicts what I've always believed, a parallel may seem preposterous, enlightening, or painful. In other words, when you draw parallels to my attention it will be a powerful human event, an important manipulation of symbols. The most important parallels will be when I've identified with someone else, most powerfully with my parents. I will often go further and *create* a parallel by co-opting my parents' manner of speech, gestures, tastes, or habits. In order to unbalance me, at strategic moments you'll address me archetypally, underlining how real and powerful such identifications are. For example, if I've been passive when my girlfriend was mean to me, and since you know my family history, you'll pointedly address me as Gerhard, my father's name: "Well, Gerhard, as always, you're very patient with Anna" (my mother).

When I was a boy, I was referred to as *Bubi*, the German diminutive often given to sons. When my first son Paul was born, I hadn't heard the word for twenty-five years, but when I picked him up, without thinking about it I said to him, "*Bubi!*" It was a powerful parallel between me and my son, a parallel unplanned and unexpected. By blurting out that word, I reassured myself that Paul was a reincarnation of me, and I also began the project of showing my son who he was. I didn't explain and say, "Your name is *Bubi*," nor did I say, "You are me"; nevertheless, that's exactly what I was saying. I've recently identified with Paul in the other direction. When I make a joke, I've noticed that I've taken to smiling ironically in just the way he smiles ironically when *he* makes a joke. More often, identifications are so much a part of us that we don't even notice that we've copied another person's ways.

A CHILD LEARNS language by being shown an analogy. This time, the analogy is between a word and the thing referred to. Over and over, parents say, "Let's put on your coat before we go out," "Where's your coat?" "Oh, look, you have a new coat, a nice red coat," or "Oh dear. Your coat is all dirty." By then the child has learned what a coat is—not an empty word he has been taught, but a living parallel between a sound and the many aspects of a coat. In other words, the child has performed a meta-psychological act, stood back from his various experiences, and said to himself, "I notice that people say *coat* a whole bunch of times and they all mean the same thing—a thing that appears in lots of places and in lots of ways." If he didn't get meta about it, he'd think there are several discrete items, all different, called *coat to put on*, *red coat*, *new coat*, and *coat that's all dirty*. The child will also have learned the rudiments of *put on*, *where is? new*, *go out*, and *dirty*. Once shown these other things repeatedly, the child will have learned that those word-sounds are also the equivalent of the thing or action being talked about, that one thing stands for another, and that it can appear in many places and in many guises. When the child announces that he sees a car, he'll say, "Car." If in response you say, "Yes, a big blue car," one day the child will repeat your new word: "Boo car." A parent doesn't give her child the definition of a word, and the psychiatrist doesn't give her patient a definition of insight. It's always about using or doing something, a human action or description rather than a simple definition.

That's why *crazy* is a word that shouldn't be censored too quickly. A child growing up has heard it many times. "Hey, stop it. That's crazy," "You little monkey, you're acting crazy again," "Look at crazy Uncle Rob making your sister laugh," "If Fred keeps doing that, he'll end up in the crazy house," or "Well, son, your mother hasn't been well. You've seen that she's been acting crazy lately, so she has to go into the hospital for a while." But if someone is called *schizophrenic*, the dozens of implications, connotations, and senses of what's going on are lost. Child or adult, the word sounds ominous and all that can be said is, "What's schizophrenia?" But everyone knows what *crazy* means—an old English word loaded with many meanings, rich and evocative, not a nasty and frightening label. This has to do with the parallels so characteristic of humans. The parallel between the word *crazy* and the person being talked about is human and understandable; the parallel between the word "schizophrenic" and the person being talked about is abstract and obscure.

So what is my point? If I say someone is crazy, you can still treat him as a full citizen and tell him to stop acting crazy; if I say someone is schizophrenic, I am conveying that he is an incomplete human being and you are silenced.

ANALOGIES ARE SURPRISINGLY familiar cultural tropes—narratives, cultural stories. You, my psychiatrist, will remind me that mine is not the only way to tell my story, that the pattern that's been discovered isn't obligatory. You'll remind me of other stories, ones that contradict what I habitually tell myself, new interpretations for old. If, for example, you notice I've repeatedly said things like "I'm a loser," you'll introduce a variant—the same topic yet sharply the reverse: "You're frightened by the idea that you have often been a winner; you feel like an imposter. You therefore constantly repeat to yourself that you're a loser." You'll have to have evidence that I am indeed a winner in certain respects, well illustrated by the Oedipus interpretation, which, because it's now a cliché, you'll talk about very cautiously.

Although alternative stories are neither right nor wrong, every and any interpretation changes the psychiatric conversation, breaks free of the earlier one. In its most banal form, the earlier conversation would have been, "I'm a loser," responded to by you with a platitude: "No you're not a loser," not to speak of more subtle versions of the despair-responded-to-with-a-pep-talk nonsense. By the way, depressives are the patients most likely to call themselves losers, but they are often smart, interesting people—winners, in other words.

Mental tricks such as finding parallels can be both disasters and good fun, the basis of puns, errors, and jokes. They also make our species uniquely successful. For example, the tides rise and fall more or less in conjunction with the moon, and many people have noticed the parallel. Other smart humans have noticed that, six to eight months after an epidemic of German measles, there is a sharp increase in birth defects in children. These discoveries have been made many times over, as was the connection between having had cowpox and immunity to smallpox. Milkmaids, who commonly got the mild disease called cowpox, were noted to be immune to smallpox, thus leading to the development of a successful vaccine. Only a creature who makes analogies could have made these important discoveries.

A jazz band plays a theme, then meddles with it. Members of the band, in turn, improvise solos, try out variations, riff on the theme—sometimes a sober repetition, sometimes a far-out variation that is barely recognizable, but we clever humans *do* recognize the parallel between the two ways of playing the theme. We also understand that the various players are bouncing off one another, conversing, having a debate and a love affair. If well done, it's sublime. A jazz orchestra does exactly what Bach and Brahms did when they wrote the *Goldberg*

Variations and *Variations and Fugue on a Theme by Handel.* All music exploits our fascination with repetition and variation, our endless need to toy with analogies. Repetition celebrates sameness; variation celebrates change, including counterpoint, changing things into their opposite. To switch examples, why have there been twenty James Bond films, all variants on the same plot, and why did Shakespeare so often write plays with a subplot that echoes the main story? We love rhyme and alliteration for the same reason. The vital human capacity for analogies is what makes the sublime possible.

DEAR PSYCHIATRIST—it's you, don't forget—as long as you stick to drawing my attention to a parallel, a resemblance, or a symbol, creating new connections, you are on safe ground. Your interpretations are additive, a supplement to my already established repertoire of associations. Once you're done with me, I won't be as narrow, will be more multilayered, more ready to look at my woes from other perspectives. Woes might not even look like woes anymore. Because your comments are unusual and unexpected, the word *supplement* isn't quite right—a good interpretation is usually interesting and sometimes thrilling, horrifying, or surprising. I could say it's a sublime experience, but I'd better not; romantics like me are ready to find things to be sublime, while others think I am preposterous and histrionic.

To add to the confusion, you'll also link episodes in my life with similar episodes in myths and fairy tales (they don't tell us how the world *was*; they tell us how the world *is*), archetypal stories that define us, links that, when you can spot them, are persuasively suggestive. This means you'll also have to wonder whether Rumpelstiltskin, Little Miss Muffet, and Cinderella are flickering in the air of this office we're sitting in. The cast of characters is bewildering; it's like a John le Carré novel. What a whirligig profession you've chosen.

> To see a world in a grain of sand
> And a heaven in a wild flower,
> Hold infinity in the palm of your hand,
> And eternity in an hour.[2]

---

2 William Blake, "Auguries of Innocence," in *The Pickering Papers*, published 1863.

As you attend to the flesh-and-blood realities of my life, you will pay close attention to the dreams I report, the games I play, the complexes I describe, and both my brilliant and idiotic actions. Like many patients, I'll be impressed at your ability to notice ordinary, seemingly trivial things that are startlingly pertinent to what's going on. Sometimes I'll overdo my admiration, at other times denigrate your performance. No matter how apparently insignificant my actions, you'll point out to me that my every one of them expresses many meanings. This superfluity dictates that you will never be dogmatic, give in to tunnel vision; the more experienced you are, the more variously you will render me real. You will take my life seriously—very seriously—as opposed to mouthing empty theoretical pronouncements such as "Everything is rooted in the social, the psychological, and the biological."

14

Sympathy or Surgery?

For this is hardest of all: to close the open hand out of love, and to be modest as a giver.
FRIEDRICH NIETZSCHE

IF I CHANGE the subject when I'm talking with a patient, I'm suggesting that what *I* am interested in is what matters, more important than what the patient is saying or doing. I'm also suggesting that I'm the boss, the conductor, and that the patient must follow my lead. I hate it when that happens; should the patient burp or giggle or yawn—or read the newspaper—he is fulfilling his part of the psychiatric bargain, putting on display who he is. Whatever he does is what's important because whatever he does teaches me about him. For example, should he neglect to mention a catastrophic event that happened yesterday, it's my job to stick to what he's actually doing, not to the catastrophe. The topic is not the secret; rather, it's his fear of telling me, his teasing (if that's what he's doing), or his fear of the topic. It's not my job to suggest that he should stop teasing, face up to the catastrophe, or fill in the details for me. For the psychiatrist, the avoidance is not a transgression but a revelation, something that in my office is more important than the catastrophe itself, just as the patient's giggle, yawn, and newspaper reading is more important than what I—or even he—might think is proper. However, if, in the middle of the appointment, the patient asks, "When did you say you'd be away?" I'll prick up my ears and keep listening, listening hard: "Hmm," I'll say, "you've changed the subject. I wonder why, all of a sudden, the topic of my being away has come up?" Only at the end of the appointment will I switch back to the literal world of administration, let go of the meta position. "Our time is up," I'll say, then add, "It's next Tuesday that I'll be away." Petty administration comes after the time is up; why the patient raises the topic of petty administration in the middle of the appointment is of interest. As he crosses the blue line, a hockey player focuses on the puck, just as the psychiatrist focuses on her patient; neither has time to think of the calendar.

Pondering fool that I am, should my patient comment on the weather I narrow my eyes and think. A cheerful greeting, acknowledgement of a black eye on my face, or praise of a painting on my wall garners only more of my pondering madness. And should the patient tell me to go to hell, fire me, or spread malicious rumours, I still don't shift, half mad with pondering. When with my patient, I forget all birthdays, decline all realities, and insist (without saying so) that what transpires in my office is exclusively artistic narrative and performance. By making only an artistic critique, I drive my patient crazy, the craziness that is the cure—if there is a cure—and which can transform him, sort of, for a moment or forever, into a work of art.

The sensitive understanding of what's going on in the minds of others is called empathy, the ability we all have to intuit the inner motives and feelings of other people. The word *empathy* is a translation from the Greek *empatheia*, and to an English speaker its meaning isn't immediately obvious. To a German speaker, the German word *Einfühlung*, which literally means "feeling into" someone else's mind and is *klar Deutsch* ("plain English"), captures the meaning beautifully. Therefore, in English, *empathy* is a tricky word, all too often because it is used incorrectly to refer to the psychiatrist's verbal or behavioural *response* to her empathic understanding of someone. The common fallacy is that the psychiatrist, in response to her new understanding, will be *sympathetic*, a response quite different from empathy. Rather, empathy refers only to any person's—in this case the psychiatrist's—ability to understand, not to her response. It's obvious that a swindler can also use empathy to understand another person, figure out who might be a vulnerable victim, a suitable prey; she empathically senses what a person thinks, and rather than reacting sympathetically or helpfully, uses what she's intuited to manipulate and cheat. Other people, nervous types, when they sense the thoughts of others, are frightened and retreat, trying not to know what they actually know.

Also fallaciously, when talking about empathy many psychiatrists highlight suffering and our appreciation of it rather than being alert to any line of thought the patient is pursuing. This emphasis also neglects empathizing deeply, figuring out the *motives* that inspire the patient's state of mind. Full understanding requires that once the psychiatrist has sensed what's going on in the patient's mind, she becomes more mentally active, struggling to understand why the patient thinks of himself as suffering, for example, or as dangerous, brilliant, or stupid. What a strong surface stance of suffering hides is never immediately obvious; hard-to-see motives are sometimes benign, other times cunning, manipulative, or cruel. Since every person is an individual, every person's motives will be different. Whoever figures out such complicated mental content can use or misuse this knowledge: the criminal can con the person, the lover can make a marriage proposal, the psychiatrist can help her patient understand himself, and the poet can write a poem based on what he's intuited.

Part of being psychologically minded is that although we don't always do it, we can think about someone else's mindset in two ways. For example, of Bobby Bruiser I can say, "He's a rotten bully," or I can ask, "What is Mr. Bruiser up to when he alienates everyone, pressures people into seeing him in a bad light, as a bully?" In other words, I can stand back and adopt a meta-psychological posture—asking "Why?" The first intuition takes bully behaviour at face value; the second intuition sees bully behaviour as a way of presenting himself, a stance that can be thought about, perhaps understood. I had a lot to say about this in chapter 11, when, instead of taking the first approach ("Marilyn Monroe is sick"), I took the second ("Ms. Monroe swindles us by portraying herself as sick—a cheat tactic that reduces the burden of being an acclaimed genius").

Empathy is fundamental—it's essential—but it would be wrong to think it is exclusively about recognizing suffering and tragedy. In the case of a patient's cruel behaviour, it can be seen as suffering only by performing a syntactic trick: changing the active voice ("He thinks and behaves sadistically") to the passive voice ("He is overwhelmed by bad impulses and thoughts")—a psychiatrist vice I often complain about. Badness in humans is thereby redefined as victimhood. I say that bad is bad, and tragedy is tragedy, and the distinction is very important.

Rather than realizing that human decency is usual, some pundits assume that the psychiatrist has, or should have, the inside track on human decency; that she is, or ought to be, more sensitive, more humane, more decent than other people. She achieves this, they say, by the use of empathy, which, when the empathizer is a psychiatrist, they seem to think has a sacred quality. Well, I'm skeptical. I doubt we psychiatrists have heavenly qualities; as far as I can tell, the community of psychiatrists has as many empathically deaf members as has any other community. Nor do I believe that empathy can be taught to everyone or that the psychiatrist can be empathic with every situation she runs into, that she can train herself to be empathic through and through. Stanley Fish doubts that anyone, through "empathy exercises," can develop an "empathy muscle."[1] Even more important is that, when she tries to understand deeply—the psychiatrist's chief assignment—and looks beneath the surface, her response to her empathic understanding is rarely automatic and intuitive, a simple sliding into her patient's mind. Instead, a penetrating intuition or deeply empathic act requires effort, intellectual work. Since all of us are biased, and since we are deeply attached to our biases, it may be impossible for the psychiatrist to put herself into the other person's shoes at all.

A skilled Israeli psychiatrist may be able to empathize with a Palestinian who advocates the end of Israel, but it's unlikely she'll be sympathetic; it's more likely she'll hate his guts. A skilled Palestinian psychiatrist may be able to empathize with an Israeli who advocates increasing the number of settlements on the West Bank, but she'd be a rare Palestinian if she sympathized with what she has come to empathically understand. These two psychiatrists could *pretend* to have sympathetic attitudes toward patients whose political opinions they find abhorrent, but patients are not fools, and most will see through fakery.

---

1 Stanley Fish, *There's No Such Thing as Free Speech: And It's a Good Thing Too* (New York: Oxford University Press, 1994), p. 217.

I hate it when, rather than understanding that empathy is a method for getting into someone else's head, these colleagues assume that empathy has a mushy quality, a family resemblance to kindness and sympathy. This is a serious misunderstanding. I'm right about this, but you should also be aware that despite my being a romantic, my scorn for psychiatric mushiness is also a madness of mine, a madness that blinds me. By now you will have realized that my choice of metaphors—rape, bullfighting, and in this chapter I add surgery—are realizations of my bias toward being a problem solver, the male thinking I will speculate about in chapter 16. This bias gives away that, like a surgeon, I think that *to save a life, it takes ... the knife*. Even though it's obvious I have a bias in favour of directness and plain talk, it's nonetheless legitimate to worry that being centred on kindness will lead the psychiatrist to neglect the problem of evil and how to talk about it. I insist that, when discerned by the psychiatric doctor, badness is not to be merely sympathized with. As she does with any other mental style or action, subtle or blatant, the psychiatrist must focus plainly on wickedness in all its nastiness—however painful this may be. Certain cancers require the surgeon to be unflinching and determined; a breast, for example, may have to be removed. Even though it is disfiguring, the surgeon mustn't shy away from doing such a surgical procedure and mustn't be mealy-mouthed: she takes action. That's what the psychiatrist must do. She is duty-bound to help the patient know himself thoroughly, including his mental cancers, and she mustn't hesitate to call a spade a spade, call evil by its name.

Soft-hearted psychiatrists, in accord with *their* craziness, will counsel the opposite. A guru who talks endlessly about empathy is often a Johnny-one-note who doesn't want to hold the patient to account for his greed, blaming, or cowardice—"hold to account" meaning "notice carefully." Such a psychiatrist can't make clear to her patient that yes, his evil side is repugnant, that this insight is ill-served if thought of as a product of victimhood—the cowardly Hitler-had-a-bad-mother explanation. Bad is bad, and wising up depends on the psychiatrist insisting that the patient face up to the unsavoury in himself, know its full awfulness. By doing that dirty job, the psychiatrist can help. If the patient blames others or implies that events in his biography or current circumstances cause him to be a bad person, the psychiatrist must be courageous and do her best to note that evil is evil, no matter what.

BECAUSE THE WORD *empathy* has lost its strict meaning, I often use the phrase *imaginative identification*, of which I discriminate two types: *modest identification* and *unflinching identification*. Modest identification is common and practical in everyday life, albeit naïve, and if she is a decent human being, the psychiatrist, like most people, will automatically respond humanely to her patient's suffering. Were we constantly unflinching, psychologizing deeply about everything ("Why did my wife say good morning when I woke up this morning?" or "Why did my friend choose to phone me at 11:43 this morning?"), we'd get nothing done.

But in the clinic, things are different. The psychiatrist *does* psychologize about everything. She knows that evil is also performance art, and that there is more to say about evil behaviour than is immediately apparent. When tackling the horrible problem of evil—it's in all of us—the psychiatrist doesn't let her patient off the hook too quickly. She hasn't done her job unless her patient repeatedly knows the fullness of his own bad nature, and if she talks too much about what her patient is fighting off—thereby implying he is a victim—she will soften, weaken, and ultimately wreck what she's trying to do. Every insight into the origins and awfulness of his bad side will tempt him to use that insight as an excuse. So what does the psychiatrist do? Well, she tries to go deeper. Through what I've called unflinching identification, she tackles the things that are hard to talk about. She calmly examines the origins of the patient's way of life, stating that biographical origins are important, but also says plainly that she fears being distracted from and losing touch with his nasty side, doesn't want to be sidetracked. She tells him, "I assume that since our job is to know you better, including your bad side, maybe especially your bad side, you probably agree with me that we've got to rub your nose in this awful stuff." (And what a dangerous metaphor *that* is! The bleeding hearts will crucify me—or will their hearts bleed for me?) And then she will carry on: "Have you more thoughts about this nastiness of yours, Mr. Smith?"

But a small number of patients prefer sympathy. When they quit—which is rare, by the way—my feelings are hurt.

15
Talking

Therapy works like a slow poison.
ANONYMOUS

THERE HAPPEN TO be several German families—Anneliese Muther (Anneliese *Henderson* Muther, whom I described in chapter 10) and her husband among them—along the road to my cottage at Horseshoe Lake. Except for Volker and Cathy Schmidt, I'm not friendly with any of them; in this country, Germans aren't tribal—or more accurately, they don't let it show that they are tribal. Because most Germans in Canada avoid history, most don't want to speak German with me, but since my German is rusty I want to practise it, so I'm annoyed when they snub my attempts to be clannish, to share a language. As well as being annoyed, I'm amused—and provoked to think. I'm a native-born Canadian, pining to speak the language of my ancestors; most of the Germans I run into are immigrants, pining to become Canadians. My attempts to speak to them are inspired by who they are; their reluctance to join in is inspired by my attempt to corrupt them, to distract them from their shaky Canadian identity, if not to derail their wish to minimize their Teutonic background. Seven decades after World War II, Germans are still touchy about history.

You may remember that in our first appointment, I noticed Mrs. Muther's language, that her diction was proper, sometimes faintly formal—although not formal enough to catch the attention of a listener less rapacious than a psychiatrist. This became clearer in later appointments. She said things like "Had I been quicker on the uptake, I'd have..." and "Were I to have commented, I'd have been..." This is a version of the conditional mood that isn't much used by English speakers (although I do use it occasionally in this book). Most people use the "if... then" version: "*If* I'd been quicker on the uptake, *then* I'd have..." and "*If* I'd commented, *then* I'd have been..."

I know why she spoke that way. When I was four (once again understanding emerges from biography, this time autobiography), my mother and I spent six months in Germany. When we got back to Canada, I'd completely lost my English, apparently couldn't speak a word. A neighbourhood child said to my mother, "Gordon can't talk!" One year later, English having been re-learned, a boy in my kindergarten class and I were in the principal's office. The other boy said something, then I said something. And I made an observation: *I speak English better than he does.* I knew absolutely that my grammar and vocabulary were, if not perfect, at a high level. Although it wasn't taught until grade one, I could read a bit, and I remember being fascinated by the peculiar, non-phonetic spelling of the word *one*—not only fascinated but thrilled. I was a kid with immigrant parents, the outsider, and I made myself an insider by urgently learning English, that thrilling language that other people spoke. Not only that, but I learned a certain style of English; I didn't speak like the roughnecks in my neighbourhood, I spoke like the kids from refined families and like my teachers. Between the ages of four and five, I'd figured out how to make it in Canada, bulldozing my way from immigrant family status to bourgeois status. Mrs. Muther's use of the conditional mood and of other highbrow grammar and diction served the same purpose. She escaped low-class status—boorish father, mother a phony—by identifying with the intellectual half of her father.

Everything we do is a matter of taste—including Mrs. Muther and I choosing to speak fancy forms of English—not to mention our personal and peculiar sexual habits, types of cowardice, and fakeries. Taste is complicated, not just a matter of following some current fashion. I have a number of interests (note that I'm treating interests, tastes, customs, habits, and styles as near synonyms), but a library wouldn't hold the list of factors that contributed to their development.

To that end, let me talk briefly about music. In my usual version of myself, I'd say that I'm moderately interested in music. My father listened to classical music, was interested in intellectual matters. Whether there was something in classical music itself that caught my interest or whether it helped me identify with my father can never be known with scientific accuracy, but by relying on analogies and other soft evidence, it's possible to say I was likely identifying with my father. What *is* a solid fact is that I needed/wanted/chose classical music as one of my preferred tastes. That interest isn't simple, nor is it mere aping of my father. I'm not just a Beethoven, Brahms, and Mozart fan; my musical interests are offbeat: Janacek, Wagner, Richard Strauss, Prokofiev. It's me, the carefully rebellious psychiatrist, uneasy about conventionality, or better, caught between Johann Sebastian Bach and Alban Berg. I doubt that I came to terms with the less conventional composers naturally. Almost certainly I worked at it—I was determined, in other words, not to be middle of the road.

My taste in music determines who I am—as do my tastes in food, clothing, posture, art, friends, habits, diction, the restaurants I choose and those I avoid, and other things not usually counted as matters of taste. My ways of being stupid, for example, are my tastes, my preferences, ways of defining myself to me and to others, as are my ways of pooping and peeing and scratching and picking at myself. Everything I do defines me. One of the difficult-to-digest conclusions I'm trying to persuade you of is that the good taste of caviar isn't in the caviar; it's in you. Good luck to the psychiatrist who thinks she can complete the job of analyzing my life. She'll have better luck counting the grains of sand on the beach here in Puerto Escondido.

Mrs. Muther again:

Meeting #4:

"What you said last time has been bothering me. But once I thought about it, it was obvious. I'm very sexual with Dan, but with Tommy, it isn't the same. And I guess I haven't told you that I started having sex when I was pretty young because I was so mature. I was twelve and got together with a fellow up at the cottage who was eighteen. Logically, I don't think it was such a big deal, but sometimes when I think of it I get very upset, thinking it might have ruined my life. I'm feeling very upset right now telling you about it. I have the idea that I drew the guy in, and actually I did because I remember him hesitating and not sure what to do. But I also hate him and still see him around at Horseshoe Lake because his family has a cottage up there too.

"My father was obsessed with me going out with guys at such a young age. He'd look out the window for me even if it was only eight o'clock. I used to purposely frustrate him by sitting in the boy's car for a while before coming in. Then he'd criticize me. But if he was drunk, he'd swear at me and call me a whore. One day we were out getting wood at the cottage and he was insulting me, so I told him I'd had sex when I was twelve years old over on the public beach. He went crazy and came after me with a stick, stabbed me with it, kept poking it into my back. But I also took care of my father, tried to help him when he'd been drinking, get him to drink lots of water when he had a hangover. I still do when we're up at the cottage."

"Remember last week?" I say. "I coughed and you asked if I was okay? Were you taking care of me too, Mrs. Muther? Anybody else you take care of?"

"Well, my husband. He's my baby. I work hard and earn more money than he does, and I take good care of our house, make nice meals for him." She pauses. "I really take care of him, do everything for him. I call him my Pasha."

I want to caricature what she's said, gently tease her about it, tell her that this sounds like a Christ story, that she seems to be a God-is-love character. This may provoke her to think—or to send me to hell. I mustn't forget that my comments are foreign, indigestible if served raw. But I'm nervy, more of a risk-taker than some. The time is almost up, but I take a chance. I'm quite calm, so my body language should tip her off that I'm not judging or criticizing her, just trying to get her thinking, get her to figure out what I mean.

"Mrs. Muther, there *is* a sort of Christlike quality to your behaviour toward your husband, don't you think? Or is it Sir Walter Raleigh flinging his cloak onto a puddle so that the sixteenth-century Queen Elizabeth wouldn't muddy her shoes?"

She frowns and looks me in the eye. Silence.

"Your father sees something else. Since men are interested in you, you are not just Christlike. He sees that you're a floozy, a *grisette*." More silence. Even though I'd caricatured her kindness and her womanliness, she has no visible reaction. After about a minute I say, "Our time is up. See you on Thursday."

"Wait. I want to ask you about what you just said. That's not quite fair. I'm in a difficult situation with my husband."

There's a bit of a pause. "Yes . . ." is all I say.

It remains to be seen how she'll handle these challenges, metaphors that are intentionally a little provocative. I want to use as many metaphors as I can—the mobile army of metaphors. And the metaphors mustn't be didactic. Like silence, metaphors are best if they are offbeat, provoke thinking. Aphorisms can serve the same destabilizing function—Pindar's "Become him who you are," for example, or the well-known Zen kōan, "We know the sound of two hands clapping, but what is the sound of one hand clapping?"

When she comes to the next meeting, Mrs. Muther is upset but in full agreement with my comments from last time, assuring me that she knows she overdoes her kindness. It seems she's decided that instead of to her husband, she'll now play second fiddle to me—that is to say, she'll quickly agree with what I say, however tentatively I've said it. Then, unexpectedly, Mrs. Muther turns into Mimi, a maiden in distress.

Meeting #5:

"You've got to help me," she says, bursting into tears. "I don't want you to tell me to leave my husband and to come back to see you only once I've done it. I'm in a mess because I'm not just involved with Dan. I'm also involved with someone else, an old boyfriend of mine from high school, whom I get together with once in a while. I'm not sure why I do these things because it just upsets me. Sometimes I can't sleep at night feeling guilty and trying to make excuses."

She pauses. "I don't know why I just said that because it's not true. I'm not involved with the fellow from high school. I just met him one day and we had a coffee. But there's something else I didn't tell you before and this is really true. Right after our honeymoon, I found out

> my *husband* was having an affair, and it was with my best friend. He's so passive that I don't know how he could get involved with someone, but he did."
>
> A long silence ensues, which I finally break. "So today you are frail and needy, must have my help, a way of defining yourself as number two in our story. Before it was your husband and father who were needy, and now it's you. And then there's the news about your husband's affair. The first affair you told about was yours, then a second one, the imaginary affair that you mentioned a minute ago, an affair that took place in Munchkin Land or somewhere. And today you tell me about a third affair, that your husband is a sinner too. It's as though his misbehaviour is less important, yours more important. But there's another possibility. Maybe you're thinking of yourself as frail today because you're getting ready to rear up and do something that's the opposite of frail, a different Jesus story, the one where he goes into the temple and throws out the moneylenders and the people selling stuff. Perhaps you're getting ready to lay down the law? Maybe your real affair and your imaginary affair are revenge, your way of laying down the law. I have an idea about that. Maybe you think that's what I want you to do, that I want you to pay your husband back. If I'm right, then you'd be going along with someone else besides your husband—this time me, going along with what you think I want you to do."

There's nothing wrong with this speech, but I'm dissatisfied. I need better analogies, better metaphors, ideas that are unusual, more evocative, more liable to puzzle her and get her thinking. If I can't find any from what I know about Mrs. Muther, I might scan my mind for a myth that fits, the stories that encode what social life is like or how we think life ought to be. It can't be one about a maternal, nurturing woman because that's what she is, so those stories won't alert her to anything (it's a cinch to find nurturing stories; there are fairy godmothers galore). I'm looking for one about a strong woman who refuses to put up with a man who doesn't act like a man, but there'd also be a problem with that because I suspect that that's exactly what she wants me to say—she senses that I want her to be strong. But I'm having trouble coming up with such a story. A scene from *Macbeth*, maybe, a strong woman who, in the face of her husband's weakness, puts her foot down:

Infirm of purpose!
Give me the daggers. The sleeping and the dead
Are but as pictures. 'Tis the eye of childhood
That fears a painted devil. If he do bleed,
I'll gild the faces of the grooms withal,
For it must seem their guilt. (2.2.51–57)

But Lady Macbeth doesn't work as a metaphor either. Once she's gone to the murder scene, she retreats—into madness. I'm having trouble finding the myth I want, one that illustrates how a woman can goad a man into action. But I have to be careful because wanting my patient to live a certain way is wanting her to satisfy *me*, my wishes—a common trap a psychiatrist can fall into. I've got to let my mind drift with this a bit, see where I'm going, follow up on a strange possibility, the possibility that myths and fairy tales are *never* about men being wimps, whiners, somatizers, hysterics, and hypochondriacs. Or is it me? Do such stories exist but my mind refuses to remember them, that I don't like the idea of a woman pushing a man around? What about Catherine the Great, who spearheaded the coup that overthrew her weak husband Peter III, Czar of Russia? A week later, co-conspirators murdered him in his jail cell. History books emphasize that Catherine was not party to the murder and, they add, when it's said that she was in on it, the stories are incorrect. Well, maybe they are, and maybe she wasn't in on the murder. But it's also possible that she *was* in on it; she certainly set the stage and made it possible. No one emphasizes *that*. Is there a bias, a skew? Is it safe to tell stories about a man laying down the law with a woman, risky to tell stories about a woman doing the same with a man? Is that why we find dominatrices funny?

These are memories of things I read about Catherine the Great years ago, and they could be distorted or just plain wrong. But does that matter? At some point I told her these thoughts and she looked at me grimly.

I'm impatient. Despite cautioning myself, I still want to get to *my* other point, *my* wish for her. *Is this all about me?* Again, I dutifully ask myself this question, but in my imagination I still want to say, *Mrs. Muther, you're so good to your husband that I'm suspicious. Your patience is over the top. I can't help wondering whether you actually want to bop him on the nose, that you're bending over backward so you won't blow your stack.*

Maybe, just maybe, you're starting to hate his guts—even though it never shows. And when I say you want to bop him on the nose, you understand that I mean you want to kill him. This imaginary comment would have been a mistake. Her cover story in which she portrays herself as submissive and Christlike in her dealings with her husband would have to give way to the same submissive story with me—discipline her husband, yes, but do it for *me*, once again going along with a man. And, of course, she'd also said that her father pushed her around.

Meeting #17:

"I don't know if it's the therapy that's doing it, but sometimes I'm impatient. The other day when I told Tommy he ought to go out to look at cars on his own, he lost his temper. And then yesterday, I screamed back. There was a yelling match and the scene deteriorated. I told him he was a useless asshole and ought to kill himself. So then he yelled back, 'Why don't you kill me, you coward. Get it over with. Do it.'" Mrs. Muther falls silent.

After a minute or so, I say, "So, the witch-Satan has shown its face, but it's not clear who it will settle on, you or Tommy. And what about the wimp-nurse? Where will it settle in?" Then I add, "Isn't it amazing that kindness and murder draw their energy from the same glands?" She narrows her eyes, takes short breaths. "Mrs. Muther, where is the deadly wife-husband, the scaredy-cat who kills?"

"Well," she says, "later that night Tommy was in bed and I was in the living room, thinking. I thought if I killed Tommy I'd be at peace, that I wouldn't have to live with my embarrassing story any more. I'd just be a plain criminal murderer. A weird idea, but that's what I thought."

"Yes," I say. "I know what it is. As long as you are Mother-Teresa-who-keeps-up-with-the-Joneses, you're at risk of being humiliated. People might find out about the fiends and angels who live in your house. But if you give up on that, become a plain criminal, it'll be a relief because you'll no longer have to be proper—you can just settle for being a murderer with nothing to hide, no more social pretensions. Sort of like your father. If you are filth, best to be without social aspirations, just be horror-filth and not have any need to worry about what other people are thinking."

Why this over-the-top language? I think it gets at a different truth. If I say marriage is difficult, I'm telling a quietly recognized truth about ordinary life, but if I wish, I can also get hyperbolic about it: "Marriage is shit." But if a marriage is actually in jeopardy, things change. Rather than fun and games, the hyperbolic truth becomes the actual truth; the jokey cast of characters now have truly taken the serious roles—demons, sadists, and thoughtless sensualists *displace* the gentler truths of everyday life. In a precarious marriage the truth is what we shouted on Halloween when trick-or-treating: "Shell out! Shell out! The witches are out." No longer exaggeration, overstatement, caricature, and hyperbole are archetypal truths, raw facts that have taken centre stage. Is there benefit in casting the Muthers as a gang of Hieronymus Bosch eccentrics? Are there other archetypal images that would work? Would the Red Queen, the White Rabbit, and the Mad Hatter be better? Daniel Craig, Pussy Galore, and Dr. No? When I comment on this menagerie, why not include farcical characters like Rangy Lil (a famous whore in the Yukon), and Mother Teresa (also known as the Overflowing Breast)?

Because I will be away next week, Mrs. Muther and I meet again the next day. She's dead set on evading what I've said, focusing instead on being the good patient who diligently and energetically fumes against her husband; it's a new project, hating her husband—because she thinks that's what I want. Because the Muses are stirring, and because Mrs. Muther is a bit off balance, I'll definitely have to change the cast of characters and introduce a new language with which to awaken her, to sidetrack her hate-my-husband "solution."

Meeting #18:

There's some talk I don't remember, which gives me a chance to tell a story, perhaps stir things up with some weird, admittedly illogical ideas about love and murder.

"Last week I watched the film *The English Patient*, Mrs. Muther. It's about love, its anguish, and the quarrelling and misunderstandings of love. Count Laszlo de Almásy (Ralph Fiennes) and Katherine Clifton (Kristin Scott Thomas) fall in love, madly and passionately, amid complications—she's married, war, national loyalties, guilt. Jealousy and the impossibility of their situation messes things up, leads to bitterness, ruptures, and reunions, anguished joys known only to those deeply in love. So, Mrs. Muther, when you plan the murder of your husband, it's a sign of love. Obviously, you've moved in the direction of what love is really like. Quarrelling is common in marriages, but it never happens with you and Tommy. Instead you've been living a fairy tale. Now that you're quarrelling, you are truly a married couple, and murder is in the air. Suffering, rage, passion, desperation—what else could it be but love?"

She is puzzled, then gives a little smile. "I can't get over you. You're always coming up with weird angles on things. You think you're so bloody smart—you *are* so bloody smart. That's why I can't imagine stopping coming here. I know what this means, that it's the fairy tale that keeps me with my husband and if I can get in touch with whatever is left of my love for him, maybe I'll be able to get over it and be able to leave him. When I wanted to kill him, it wasn't just a sign that I could see him as a real person. It was me getting ready to leave him, or at least thinking about leaving him or at least stopping catering to him, changing the stupid chemistry of what's going on."

As I must, when she tells me I'm smart, I treat her words as data, something else to be analyzed and get me back on track, silently making a meta-commentary to myself about what she says. But I'm also flattered, happy to know she recognizes my brilliance, my power, my heroic masculinity. The worst thing about the psychiatric job is that our patients admire us, sometimes love or worship us, and whether we admit it or not, when they speak well of us we have trouble staying meta. Even as we know it's ridiculous nonsense, we believe what they say, a major source, perhaps *the* major source, of psychiatric error. When I'm not firing on all cylinders, I'm sure I encourage her admiration, perhaps with my body language, subtly cheering her on when she lists her husband's faults, doing soul-murder for her. There are hints that I'm Mrs. Muther's ally in the dirty project of making her husband irrelevant.

"Yes," she says. "I'm supposed to murder him and yes, he's supposed to kill himself. Damn it all—you ought to kill my husband for me. What's a girl supposed to do, and what's this helpless female stuff I'm getting into? Ordinary life is weird, weirder than I realized.

Why have you let me go down this path for so long without drawing this stuff to my attention? I've told you nothing about my childhood or about my mother and her bitch sisters who constantly criticized their husbands. You've always been so bloody polite about me not telling, which makes me wonder whether you're some kind of a pansy or something. My sexual problems are probably because my parents never taught me what was what. How was I supposed to know how to behave when sex was always this big secret around the house?"

She falls silent, and after a minute or so my mind starts jumping around. Something is coming into focus, a poem about how much we know without knowing how we know it. I wait a bit longer and then, without explanation, say:

I've never been to Scotland,
I've never seen the sea,
Yet I know how heather looks
And what a billow be.

She waits for me to elaborate but I don't say a word, not even that it is a poem by Emily Dickinson.

In ancient Athens, the worst thing about being ostracized was no longer having freedom of speech: not to say what one thought was, to the Greeks, the way of a servant. Frankness, a characteristic of aristocrats, became, under democracy, secularized into free speech. Once we've obtained free speech, most people agree that it's criminal to squander it, even when speaking up is risky. Therefore, I wonder, am I too patient and quiet? Do I refrain from pointing out the benign way she tells an awful story, that she is as passive as her husband? Do I say to her clearly that both she and her husband are hiding their heads in the sand as their marriage goes sour? Even though I think I'm tough and bold, my descriptions strike me as too subtle: when I speak of her and her husband's passivity, I am circumspect, careful, speak in euphemisms and circumlocutions. Fake courtesy and discretion, in other words. Maybe—how to know for sure?—I could tell Mrs. Muther a story about the bullfighting I've seen in Mexico City to illustrate what's going on.

In the *plaza de toros*, a demand is placed on us to acknowledge the equal status—full citizenship, so to speak—of both bull and matador. (I know, of course, that in the bullfight, equal citizenship is a myth, but it is an artistic performance that teaches us about the idealistic, hoped for equality of bull and matador, of man and woman, of prime minister and every other citizen.) "The bull and matador love each other," I could say, emphasizing that it is a *real* love, a story of demands, anguish, frustration.

IN THE MEANTIME, something else is in the air. If a man and a woman, a psychiatrist and his patient, meet alone in a comfortable room—couch, easy chairs, dim lighting—carefully examine serious life issues, and talk intimately and personally, something else comes up. I've received an email from Mrs. Muther. There is no message, only Shakespeare's sonnet 138:

> When my love swears that she is made of truth
> I do believe her, though I know she lies,
> That she might think me some untutored youth,
> Unlearned in the world's false subtleties.
> Thus vainly thinking that she thinks me young,
> Although she knows my days are past the best,
> Simply I credit her false speaking tongue:
> On both sides thus is simple truth suppressed.
> But wherefore says she not she is unjust?
> And wherefore say not I that I am old?
> Oh, love's best habit is in seeming trust,
> And age in love loves not to have years told.
> Therefore I lie with her and she with me,
> And in our faults by lies we flattered be.

By sending the email, Mrs. Muther is taking a page from my book, quoting Shakespeare, whom I probably mention too often. But she's also announcing an achievement, recognizing another part of talking-cure dilemma deeply and thoroughly, familiarizing herself with how complicated life is, seeing the endlessly complex relations between a man and a woman. She's not indulging in the get-rid-of-symptoms cure. Instead, she's getting a glimpse of the life-is-complicated cure, the there-are-moral-predicaments-everywhere cure. Having given up on the hope that she can resolve dilemmas, Mrs. Muther has assigned herself a new job: *exploring* dilemmas.

Shakespeare's sonnet says explicitly that "... age in love loves not to have years told / Therefore I lie with her and she with me," so it seems clear that Mrs. Muther is thinking about us going to bed together. When she next comes in I'll have to find a way of making this email teach us something. What evocative images might I conjure up? I could perhaps try out delirious mad love and similar romantic language, or I could go toward *floozy* and *grisette* again. *Whore* would certainly be too ugly. Or maybe I could get worthy love and fuck-for-the-sake-of-fucking into the same sentence? Or maybe I should ask her about me, how I've been in on this turn of events, how I might have promoted it, wanted love and lovemaking to exist in the office (anyone who is surprised or shocked by this isn't paying attention to life). I'll see tomorrow what mood she's in, what cues she's giving off, and it'll come clear what I should say.

Such a fantasy invitation isn't offered without having received signals from the invitee, signals from me that I would welcome it, the promise that, since Tommy Muther is a write-off, she and I, without thinking it explicitly, are really Anneliese and Gordon, and more—much more. Of course I show Mrs. Muther my muscles—subtly—making sure she sees my interpretive abilities, even though in the foreground I'm only diligent and professional. I've boned up on how to do the psychiatric version of the sexual game and do it so slyly that, unless I pay extra close attention, I don't even know I'm doing it. I always do it, and always will—just as every psychiatrist does his or her version of it. But don't forget that the patient, in this instance Mrs. Muther, is not innocent. You'll have seen how she pressures me into thinking of her as the princess who needs rescuing, inviting me to be her hero. I know our private, secret agenda, and so does she, although she doesn't know it as glibly as I do.

But as you'll see, when she arrives, she's upset about something else. It is March 2012.

Meeting #20:

"The other day you said I was hoarding all the virtue in my marriage, letting my husband be the less worthy person, the weak needy guy. I haven't been able to stop thinking about it. I'm so helpful that he can't help but feel guilty. But I think it's worse than you said. I thought that that's how I'm punishing him for being so passive, being nicer and nicer to him, that I'm doing the death-by-a-thousand-cuts on him instead of honestly telling him what's bothering me. Kind of a sadistic glee in sticking it to him. But I'm also mad at you. You keep stirring things up, and I keep getting kinder and kinder with Tommy. And I'm always so agreeable with what you say.

"But there's something else. I'm really upset about it," she goes on. "Over the last few days I've been reading about the Tori Stafford case in the newspapers."

Eight-year-old Tori Stafford had been raped and murdered, and Michael Rafferty was on trial for the crime. His girlfriend, Terry-Lynne McClintic, already convicted of the crime, had testified for the prosecution about what had happened. She had kidnapped Tori Stafford for her boyfriend, she said, and accompanied him to a remote place where he raped the child. She also testified that, before the rape, she had purchased green garbage bags and a hammer, and that afterward, she had put a bag over the child's head and killed her with the hammer. "I can't tell you how upsetting it is reading about this case," Mrs. Muther said. "That woman did it for her boyfriend, and it's driving me crazy because I'm like that, always doing things for Tommy."

I'm taken aback and stay silent for two or three minutes. "Yes," I say. "I see your point. I've got a thought about all this. Listen, I think we can put it together like this: You and I are co-conspirators. We've made a pact, decided that when you and I speak ill about your husband's passivity, we're speaking in code. In truth I've been having a wonderful time raping you and stealing you away from your husband, and you, evil wife, are delighted at our game—except it's too serious to call it a game. We're quite a pair, we two, because it's obvious we're slowly and methodically killing Tommy Muther, fixing him, grinding him down until there's nothing left of him."

I stay silent as she looks at me wildly. "Oh no," she says.

"Yes, you've figured it out. You are the woman who does things for men, including me, so when today's appointment is done, you are to stop off at the hardware store, buy green garbage bags and a hammer. And you are to finish what we have been doing to Tommy, and do it for me, on my behalf, for my pleasure."

She has made the interpretation, has revised her own story yet again; I have put her insight into words and fed it back to her.

"My God," she replies, tears streaming down her face. "I can't believe this. This is what we've been leading up to. I can't believe it. That's why I can't read about the Tori Stafford case. I always thought I was a nice person."

Mrs. Muther had stumbled on an unexpected reality, a nasty reality. Such a eureka moment impresses both patient and psychiatrist, bowls us over. After that, Mrs. Muther became cautiously different. Once a rescuer, she was now dallying with new interpretations of herself and her situation, caught up in her own mind. She was in a state of half autism, letting go of the nasty embeddedness of her old way of life, now facing inward, watching, wising up, her version of *The Magic Mountain,* a world where minutes, days, and years don't matter, and things unfold as they will. I have entered her life as a doctor, but that idea too has become unclear. Mrs. Muther and I are in a war as well as a tango, a love affair as well as a pissing contest, and—a metaphor that's a bit more of a stretch—the sublime problem of seeing that Mrs. Muther and I are performers in a bullfight.

Meeting #24:

"I must have hated that good-for-nothing father of mine too, him with all his intellectual baloney. You do that intellectual stuff too. I've never mentioned it, but every time you talk about Greek myths and stuff like that, I'm annoyed. Probably want to kill you too—hah!"

She is right. I'd started out with intellectual baloney in the first appointment, finding a way to mention Nietzsche.

A long pause.

"My mother and her sisters always criticized men, especially their husbands and brothers, but none of them criticized my father. They let him off the hook because he went to university, and they thought they were supposed to respect him."

Both she and I are silent for a long five minutes.

"Yeah, I'm like my mother and her sisters. I'm kind to Tommy all the time, as though he's special. I'm walking through my mother's marriage, step by step. Just as it took a while for me to see that my marriage was wrong, my mother probably didn't see what was going on in her marriage at first. That doesn't mean I'm leaving Tommy. I have to think a bit more about all my messing around. I always thought my mother wasn't promiscuous like me, except that now that I think about it, I'm not 100 percent sure of that. I'll have to think about it. I always think of her as so sweet and pure, but there's got to be more to her than that. If she was a bad wife in some way, maybe I'm being bad because that takes the spotlight off her so I can keep thinking she's such a great mother. Come to think of it, she was careless with me, let me hang around with that eighteen-year-old guy who was way too old for me." She stops and giggles. "And you are way too old for me.

"My mother and her sisters didn't just criticize their husbands. None of them acted like women. They all acted like boards, sort of beefy and square. My mother was never an example for me for how to be a woman—she walked around in baggy clothes and bare feet—but my father was a nice-looking man."

I hesitate, then say, "What you're telling me, Mrs. Muther, is that your mother left the responsibility for womanliness in your home up to you. And you did take on that role. You became an attractive and sensual woman at a young age, yet your mother didn't do her duty and act like a model of femininity and sexiness for you. I remember you told me that your mother wanted you to be a cheerleader at school. It seems she was to be a dud and you were to be the sexy girl in the family. You did it, too, became what she wanted, but you added something else—you made sure you got bad feedback about your womanliness. Remember how you told your father that you had sex on the beach when you were twelve years old? You made sure he had awful thoughts about you. You were doing the same thing when you used to sit outside the house in the car when you had a date and made sure your father noticed you were out there. He called you a whore. Now that I think of it, you even got me to call you a grisette. I think I used the word grisette to avoid using the word whore."

Like many patients, Mrs. Muther decided that the end of June would be natural time to end our work. (What ritualized creatures we are! We think we are still school children.) Some will think that Mrs. Muther and I ought to have discovered shocking or sublime truths, things essential, special, or eternal. Others will wonder what happened to her marriage and to Dan, her lover. (The answer? I don't know.) Right to the end, she tended to think that what we did was special (as did I, in my heart of hearts), but in truth it was not, and she and I talked about her idealization of me and of our work often enough that she became somewhat immunized against this folly, and against mine. We had a series of insights under our belts, intuitions that were analogies, how one idea stands in for or displaces another and how several ideas are condensed into one. Such practices are common in the offices of talking doctors, but in another era, in the future, it will be different. Instead of modernism, Samuel Beckett, and deconstruction, it will be a psychiatric wisdom or a psychiatric tyranny as yet unknown.

By taking up residence in a different place (metaphorically speaking), Mrs. Muther has created a void, and the place in which she once lived—and still does, some of the time—is now depleted. She is well aware of this, thinks to herself, Oh, that's what I used to do, used to believe in. Or she may treat the void as though it is something real and substantial, something to be dealt with, to be crafted into a romantic catastrophe. ("Holy Jesus, man, looks as though life has no more meaning. What do I do now?") Contrariwise, she may turn her loss of the past into a romantic achievement, awe-inspiring and extraordinary. ("How amazing. This is the real truth. Wow—the Void!") In any case, she will have changed, expanded her interiority, the range of her aloneness.

Notice the impact of this fragment of Louise Glück's poem "Prism." Reading it, our own loneliness takes hold and at the same time is alleviated—both an awful insight and a cure.

> A night in summer. Sounds of a summer storm.
> The great plates invisibly shifting and changing—
> and in the dark room, the lovers sleeping in each other's arms.
> We are, each of us, the one who awakens first,
> who stirs first and sees, there in the first dawn,
> the stranger.[1]

---

1 Louise Glück, "Prism," in *Averno* (New York: Farrar, Straus, Giroux, 2006).

Change isn't a product of remembering things or of accomplishing popular cures—including resolving conflicts, connecting with one's true self, mindfulness, maturing, or achieving sexual genitality (as a psychoanalyst might put it). Change isn't about *accomplishing* anything. Rather, it's about grappling and fiddling with the inevitable—things like aloneness, triumph, guilt, and how to teach juniour to tie his shoelaces. In Mrs. Muther's case, it was her magical belief that she was or could be an ultimately kind and generous person.

Published reports of psychotherapy "cures"—all other psychiatric "cures" too—are always suspect. Every psychiatrist has dramatic cures on record, cures that can happen within days, sometimes after years-long crippling unwellness. Only the uninformed public and naïve and credulous psychiatrists think such cases are examples of real change. Mrs. Muther was more ordinary, her story only partly coherent, the events of her treatment mundane, the outcome indeterminate. As James Joyce put it, "I am quite content to go down to posterity as a scissors and paste man," which is to say that the treatment, like life, is the creation of a collage, a collage being a way of putting a life together, less smoothed out than when we translate our lives into a traditional story or a miracle-worker story. A new collage takes the place of the collage that wasn't working. If the results of a treatment are remarkable and dramatic instead of incoherent, puzzling, and indeterminate, I suspect it's someone's fancy rather than real change.

AS WE'VE SEEN, cultural subgroups are tribes—solidarities, interpretive communities—and all of us sign on with many. We pick the interpretive communities that suit us, ways of life we think will put us into categories that seem best. A style judged by someone to be best can be familiar or peculiar to others—crook, failure, fool—but all are tribal categories with whom we can establish a solidarity.

What Mrs. Muther switched to was an unfamiliar, alien interpretive community, an intrusion into what she'd imagined of herself, a bit of culture shock, especially because she'd spent so much of her life being a genteel-lady-with-a-secret-dark-side, not an outsider immigrant, and not white trash like Michael Rafferty and Terry-Lynne McClintic. And a bit of culture shock is what the talking doctor wants. I, an Anglophone

Canadian, had such a culture shock a few days ago, in a mini-panic when I had to ask for a cheeseburger in Spanish—I don't speak a word—in the crowded chaos of a fast-food joint here in Mexico City. *Drama, disquiet*, and *embarrassment* are words that emphasize that culture shock has an impact.

I, the open-minded psychiatrist, have opinions, believe there are bad stories after all, stories that limit my patients. These stories flourish in all of us.

- Women are bitches or idiots or both.
- Men are brutes or wimps or both.
- Americans (Jews, Muslims, immigrants, liberals, conservatives, blacks, whites) are ruining the world.
- Every day, in every way, the world is getting better and better.
- Every day, in every way, the world is getting worse and worse.

Since these are storylines, hence neither true nor false, I am happy to both believe and disbelieve them. To this absurdity, the only sensible response is bewildered amusement, a state that can't be avoided in life.

With people who avoid the logic loved by scientists, especially those who are flamboyant and histrionic—Anna O., Kim Kardashian, Arnold Schwarzenegger, and me once in a while—it seems a bit of logic would be the order of the day. But I have a hunch I'm wrong, that drama may still be a necessary medicine, drama that matches the histrionics of the hysteric blow for blow. Yet I also have a lingering hunch I'm wrong about this—that emphasizing drama is my simplistic hope that I can find something to hang my hat on, still hoping for a clear explanation of how someone is "cured."

New stories may be unnerving, but they offer opportunities, including the unpleasant but obvious opportunity to realize that the original idea the patient had in mind, the cure he'd hoped for, was ridiculous, like thinking there is a cure for life. Even though it's not really a cure, the patient will have achieved something, the thing called insight, held as an ideal by many people, first heard about by Westerners when we read about Socrates's notion that the unexamined human life is not worth living. But what if self-examination is just intellectual baloney? This ideal is present in lots of other religious and philosophical writing, for example, Laozi (Lao Tzu): "The sage, because he confronts his problems, never has any." His conclusion is, of course, ridiculous.

Once the psychiatrist has interested her patient in a series of new metaphors about his life, the patient will tell new stories, ones that will make him smile, snarl, or weep about his previous ways of understanding things. There's no explaining why we now prefer and find sublime the metaphor of the Oedipus complex— in other words, metaphors about sexual, marital, and family problems. It's just the way we talk about people nowadays. Nor do we know how Freud came up with these ideas—he would have said his patients told them to him—popularized, and propagandized so many of these ways of putting the world together.

The centrepiece of a psychiatric relationship is curiosity, the never-ending determination to treat human behaviour as a performance that can be decoded. The psychiatrist endlessly analyzes and invites her patient to join in. Although polite, the psychiatrist's inquisitiveness is unremitting, not because she won't rest until she finds the answer, but because she knows there is no answer, that she'll never finish discovering new and interesting angles on what her patient is revealing.

PART FOUR

THINKING

16

A Guide for the Sexually Perplexed

Of the delights of this world, man cares most for sexual intercourse, yet he has left it out of his heaven.
MARK TWAIN

LOVE AND HATE get stirred up in the psychiatrist's office—not just in maidens in distress, men in need, gays and lesbians forlorn, but also in psychiatrists despondent at being maligned, and in every kind of lover, persecutor, or victim. The kaleidoscope of roles women and men adopt needs attention, but since this is social speculation rather than science, all I offer is an invitation to think. When I insist that my arguments are speculations, and when I remind myself that self-doubt and self-questioning are important, I'm the psychiatrist with both feet planted firmly in mid-air, one of the necessary personas of the psychiatrist, the one I hate to take on, yet who I must be if I'm to think like a psychiatrist. My argument will include the ideas that men do their duty, rev up their Ferraris, shoot guns, and solve problems while women contemplate mysteries, suffer from the vapours, and hold the world together.

Now that there are many women psychiatrists, I've been hoping that, rather than endlessly wanting to "solve" problems in the style of men, women's voices might influence my profession to be more contemplative. But it hasn't happened; instead, whether a woman or a man, we psychiatrists are in a rut, endlessly thinking our job is to be enlightenment rationalists, to come to logical conclusions about our unhappy patients. Just the same, because mystery is the province of women, paying attention to womanliness may lead us in a different direction, looking inward at the world of darkness and ambiguity, of sensuality and guilt. The following story, silly but profound, demonstrates the difference between a problem and a mystery.

Some problems are easy to solve—for example, how to get over a wall. The answer: lean a ladder against the wall, climb the ladder, stand on top of the wall, and jump down to the other side. The problem of the penis is also simple: does it stand up or does it not stand up? Does it squirt or does it not squirt? If not, pop a Viagra. And that's about it. It's all about clarity, and when we've solved such a problem, we use the sense of vision as a metaphor: "I see," we say.

A woman's genitals are another matter. They're complicated and tucked away, never clearly seen. Dark and mysterious, the vagina has secret nooks and crannies, unknown even to women. Because it has an ambiguous smell, when a man leaves the bed of love, he may groan with happiness, revel in the fact that he is saturated with femininity—and take a shower. It's a tricky topic, one men skate around, make jokes about while drinking beer. The nervous ribaldry is evidence that we're dealing with something unsettling, a mystery. Because mysteries are ambiguous, we use the sense of smell as a metaphor: "There's something fishy," we say. Men's genitals also have an ambiguous smell, but even if we notice this, we don't make jokes about men's sexual smells. This is part of the mystery.

I would add that woman-think, the underpinning of wisdom, is allied to artistic thinking, although if there are more women artists than men, I haven't noticed. Nevertheless, the allusive thinking of the artist is more linked to mysteries than to solving problems. And when Marilynne Robinson shows me how to do it in her novel *Gilead*,[1] I learn from her:

> My grandfather's grave turned into the light, and the dew on his weedy little mortality patch was glorious.

---

1 Marilynne Robinson, *Gilead* (Toronto: HarperCollins, 2004), p. 209–10.

"'... weedy little mortality patch'—how fine that is," says James Wood of this passage. In his book *The Nearest Thing to Life,* Wood calls Robinson's account "noticing"—what I've called watching and describing. The title[2] points to the same way of observing, the style of both the critic and the psychiatrist. Artistic ecstasies take many shapes, especially if I expand the definition of the word *artistic.* Because Marilynne Robinson is seriously religious, I want to say that thinking about God is an artistic ecstasy for her, but also that every romantic love is kin to artistry, as is finding characters like Arnold Schwarzenegger sexy (to some people). Also, the delicate grace of modesty and remembering sitting on the Zócalo of San Cristóbal de las Casas on New Year's Day.

The vagina is also—sort of—the site of orgasms, although because I'm a man, therefore destined to be an enlightenment rationalist, I'm supposed to be physiologically accurate and say that the clitoris is the site of orgasms. Despite rationalism, some female orgasms are obvious, others enigmatic, small or large, and sometimes vague enough that one can't tell where, when, or whether an orgasm has happened. Because such things can't be learned from books or lectures, and because young men squirt at the drop of a hat, they know little about this orgasmic kaleidoscope; it is crucial information that must be learned from a woman. These are not stands-up-doesn't-stand-up propositions or matters of squirt-squirt—things that are only boring; it's the revolutionary idea that love and life can be learned about only through darkness and ambiguity. Another way of saying this is that there are two kinds of orgasms, two ways of thinking about psychiatry, two kinds of lives. The first is fulfilling a wish, perhaps a biological accomplishment like an ejaculation. The second is the life of desire, fulfilling even though desire is insatiable and given to us by the gods rather than by our physiology.

Don't get me wrong: maleness and penis-pride are important. They guarantee that men will protect tribe and family, will impose the rules that allow society to work. Women learn the lessons of the penis from men, just as men learn the lessons of the vagina from women. A consequence is that when a woman is afraid of a man, she fears he will

---

2 James Wood, *The Nearest Thing to Life* (Waltham, Massachusetts: Brandeis University Press, 2015).

rape her; when a man is afraid of a woman, he fears her mysteries, her female sexuality—"What do women want?" he asks.

The importance of the vagina (and the clitoris and the orgasm and women) is that they lead us into the strangeness of the world that makes life worth living, states of rapture that, in human affairs, take priority over being rational. These vital matters can't be taught in a classroom or read about in a book; men have to learn about these matters through love, murmurs, and subtle hints: pillow talk isn't just giggling. When Siegfried and Brünnhilde meet behind a barrier of fire, they are innocents, but they quickly learn that lovemaking isn't just sex: Brünnhilde teaches Siegfried the secrets of intuition; he teaches her about power. Unless enlightened by a woman, a man thinks in the language of power, that the bullfight is a murder (don't forget that I'm in Mexico and have recently been to the *plaza de toros*), something to laugh about after having a few drinks, a nasty form of my squirt-squirt metaphor.

Why does this matter? It's because the job of the psychiatrist is to help her patient to see that she and he are faced with two issues: unending moral dilemmas and human self-deception, topics only properly addressed once both patient and doctor have studied every novel, consulted every seer, and analyzed every myth. Should she fail to take seriously my metaphor of what patient and doctor should read and study, the psychiatrist would be a fool, would believe that her patient's problems can be solved rather than being pondered.

The psychiatrist I'm worrying about is a reincarnation of Ludovico Settembrini, a character in *The Magic Mountain*. Through Settembrini, Thomas Mann (politely) caricatures the Western European celebration of democracy, or more specifically, the West's emphasis on worldly freedom and the outer freedoms achieved in a democracy, as distinct from the darker and more personal interests of Central and Eastern European intellectuals. The freedom of the West, Settembrini argues, is full of life and optimism—"problems can be solved"—as opposed to the freedoms preferred by Germans and Russians, the darker, more pessimistic freedoms of those who think about the inner life, ambiguity, the navel of things. In the metaphors I used when I introduced this subject, this dichotomy is also caricatured: I called it male thinking and female thinking.

UNLIKE OTHER DOCTORS, a psychiatrist sees only one patient each hour, so a missed appointment is a financial blow. North American talking doctors insist this problem must be solved according to the lights of Western society. They therefore have two clear solutions: one group of psychiatrists imposes a contract that charges for missed appointments, even when the patient takes a vacation. The second group does *not* charge for missed appointments, instead choosing the riskier small business approach. Both billing options avoid a dispute over money.

If an important part of the psychiatrist's job is to help her patient explore moral dilemmas, why the devil would she sidestep a moral dilemma over money? My answer is that psychiatrists who do this—almost all psychiatrists—are enthralled by the idea that, through logic, the world can be made pure and clean, are hoping upon hope that linear thinking can solve all problems. I think otherwise; I want my patients to be thoughtful, note that life is endlessly complicated, rarely pure and clean. My practice is to try to think like a dark-minded Eastern European, like Dostoevsky and Kafka: if my patient misses an appointment, by not explaining my billing practices and leaving things uncertain, I make life difficult for both the patient and me. Obviously, if the patient's wife dies, I won't bill him for his missed appointment; if he's in a hotel room with his secretary at our appointment time, I *will* bill him. But most of the time it's not so simple. The atmosphere I try to create is this: "There's money at stake; who should take the loss? A decision is needed, and it's a tough one, sometimes impossible. It's actually a mystery, not the province of manhood; womanly thinking is called for. But be careful. If you fall in love with darkness and ambiguity there is a risk: your thinking can become so convoluted that you could disappear up your own darkness.

Woman's power to illuminate mysteries is a secret. Tiresias, who in his lifetime had been both a man and a woman, revealed the truth, that a woman has nine times more pleasure in love than a man, a secret so terrible that Hera blinded him for his indiscretion. The ancients had long known all this. Men, they said, take action: rape, kill monsters, fight battles, shoot arrows. Hesiod informs us that only women have *mêtis*—wisdom—so when Zeus wanted to personally give birth to

Athena, the goddess of wisdom, he derived the wisdom from Mêtis, his first wife, by swallowing her, acquiring the wisdom that transforms barbarism into civility.

MANY WOMEN HIDE their intelligence (think Diane Keaton, Judy Holliday). My suspicion is that because many men are shy or uncomfortable around smart women, women try to not pose a threat, to not stir up a touchy subject, aware that boyfriends and husbands hate it if their woman is right and they are wrong. "Women's science," someone called it. Some women are extreme about this tactic. They adopt some version of hysteria that, from one point of view, is giddy or silly, and from another point of view, is wonderfully feminine. But hysteria is a bad word, and if I try to rehabilitate it, I'll fail. In the Western world, it's now uncommon for a woman to swoon or have the vapours, but women still shriek at the sight of a mouse, and some pass out when Justin Bieber shows up. It's a generous and politically wise tactic, the ploy of making herself desirable by portraying vulnerability—not acting like a coward or a wimp, but like a woman.

A woman might, on the other hand, act like the young woman in the dive shop I was in this morning here in Puerto Escondido. She and the boss were debating in Spanish about the scuba equipment I should be issued, uncertain about what my 170 pounds was in kilos. As they debated, the young assistant, probably still in her teens, held my arm under the sleeve of my T-shirt, apparently unaware that I might find this unusual. In fact, I liked both the touch and the chance to think about a cultural difference, but it also made me nervous. It was a culturally appropriate friendliness that in Toronto would be forward or slutty—for the greatest fools, sexual harassment. An apocryphal story is told in which Nietzsche, having been tricked into going into a brothel, nervously plays the piano. Esmeralda, one of the women, stands beside him as he plays and puts her hand on his arm, a touch that possessed him violently enough that he pursued her, became infected, and eventually died of syphilis—died because of a touch.

I remember, too, walking on a dusty road in Vietnam, when a woman of fifty or so silently walked up beside me, hooked her arm into mine, and walked with me. After walking three or four hundred metres, just as silently, she went on her way. We didn't have a common language, so no words were exchanged. My guess? Hospitable behaviour toward a foreigner.

The words *tactic* and *portrayal* make it clear that when I talk about how women hide their strengths, I'm insisting that these are purposeful actions, not things innate or natural to women. Men, in complement, can then portray themselves as heroes who rescue maidens, drown unwanted kittens, and shoot groundhogs. In the case of men, being a bully-boy, smart, or athletic (can hold his liquor, throw money around, tell of exploits, enthuse about the hum of a BMW engine, assertive manner, etc.) may seem as pointless as being a helpless female—except that these male and female performances really do have a point, a vital and inspiring point. All are announcing pivotal social practices: men are rational, competitive, action oriented; women are nurturing, wise, social network creators—each gender role vital. Were we to homogenize them, we'd end up with Pablum, platitudes, the pallid, and the humdrum; the golden mean is boring. I suggest Marilyn Monroe and Clint Eastwood as once-in-a-while role models. Under other circumstances, choose Madame Curie (the first person to win two Nobel prizes) and Albert Einstein as role models, but aren't Marilyn and Clint more fun?

The need to elevate the man is an obvious element in hysteria. The classical "Eek, eek!" young woman, the one who swoons, and who conforms to the hated-by-feminists image of the giddy female, has method in her madness; her style serves a purpose: "I'm helpless and a bit silly, so you big, heroic men have to help me." The YouTube video series, *Sh*t Girls Say*, is a parody of female expressions and behaviours that illustrate my point better than would a thousand words. Don't get me wrong; men have complementary hyper-masculine habits that are analogous to what hyper-feminine women do: bully-boy talk, drinking too much, fighting, swearing—at its worst, killing, rape, torture, and pillage. Waging war on crimes is important, but good luck to anyone who thinks we can eradicate masculine behaviours, especially since some of these behaviours are heroic and desirable; some archetypes are intractable. I assume that the ghosts of Norman Mailer and Ernest Hemingway are in gleeful approval of the men in this German *Wirtschaft* (inn), while Arthur Schopenhauer's ghost—such a snob—disapproves:

> Schopenhauer had dinner at the Englischer Hof, where every day he entertained the same ritual. He would place a gold coin on the table, only to recover the coin before leaving. An indignant waiter lusting after the coin for himself inquired about the significance of this ritual. Arthur answered that it was the silent outcome of a wager he had made with himself—he would leave the gold coin in the poor box if the gentlemen at that inn would speak of anything else but horses, dogs, or women.[3]

If men are boors, this means they are rough and tough and strong. This includes the idea that they must participate in the maiden-in-distress complex, both sexes keen on the image of heroic men who save troubled damsels. But it's easy to realize that most men are equally ready to embrace the idea that women should prop them up, devote themselves just as enthusiastically to a Vulnerable-Man Complex, the perfect complement to the maiden complex, even propping up men who, on the surface, appear to be strong. Superman and Spiderman, for example, are male heroes who have to be saved by women worshipping them, overlooking their foibles, ignoring the truth about men, about the befuddled Clark Kent, incapable of recognizing Lois Lane's womanliness, and Peter Parker, regularly in a mess with Mary Jane. (I hear that in the end he marries her.)

Some female patients worry that their husbands, boyfriends, or fathers are not manly enough; some male patients worry that they aren't as manly as they ought to be. For fear of assassination, I haven't said it bluntly, but I will now: *all* my patients, men and women alike, worry about the weakness of men, which I announce because part of me believes what I've just said, and also because such a belief comforts me. If true, it will nail down a solid truth for me, an eternal truth—something, anything—that once and for all I can hang my hat on. Despite such anxious mental shenanigans, the weak man is an archetypal idea: James Bond is a vain adventurer; cowboys always fall for the demure preacher's daughter. Thackeray's *Vanity Fair* makes this explicit in its

---

3 Dale Jacquette, *The Philosophy of Schopenhauer* (London and New York: Routledge, 2015), p. 266.

subtitle: *A Novel without a Hero*; all of the novel's male characters are pathetic non-heroes. And, says Thackeray:

> I know few things more affecting than that timorous debasement and self-humiliation of a woman. How she owns that it is she and not the man who is guilty: how she takes all the faults on her side: how she courts in a manner punishment for the wrongs which she has not committed, and persists in shielding the real culprit! It is those who injure women who get the kindness from them—they are born timid and tyrants, and maltreat those who are humblest before them. (chapter 50)

Wagner's weak heroes? Tristan (a mortal wound), Siegfried (a vulnerable back), Amfortas (an agonizing wound that won't heal). Homer's damaged men? Oedipus (a swollen foot), Hephaestus (crippled), Achilles (a vulnerable heel), Philoctetes (a stinking wound on his foot). Who else? The answer is easy: Jesus was wounded, the men reading this are wounded, I am wounded. It's a bit harder, but these stories can be retold to illustrate the opposite: the weakness of women, another tempting "truth."

Sinuous figures of men and women, sinuous columns, and sinuous furnishings embellish the art deco Palacio de Bellas Artes in Mexico City. I was there some years back to watch a celebration of manhood and womanhood—flamenco. The principal man was good, did all the steps and made all the moves, including sinuous moves, but something was missing. Although all the women were fabulous—scornful, maddening, smoulderingly mysterious—as the afternoon went on, subtle gestures gave away that this particular man was not proud enough—not *arrogantly* proud enough—of his masculinity. A few weeks later, back in Toronto, I was still frustrated. The man had disappointed me; I want heroic masculinity intact and perspicuous. I got out an old videotape (now it's on YouTube) and watched José Greco do, in black and white, what I'd missed in Mexico City, manhood and talent untarnished.

Freud's first patients were hysterics, and when I studied psychiatry, we—mostly men—were required to follow sacred rules: like Freud, we were to take on a hysterical woman as our first patient, even though then, as now, hysterical patients were hard to find. In collusion with our teachers, we picked a woman from the waiting list who had, or who we imagined had, hysterical "features." Hysteria did exist, of course, but such patients rarely came to the clinic. As they do now, and as they did in the days of Jean-Martin Charcot in Paris, and Sigmund Freud and Josef Breuer in Vienna, they went to neurologists, complaining of pains, paralyses, visual problems, twitches, fits. Nowadays, as well as seeing neurologists, these patients seek out pain doctors—especially pain doctors—and are liable to be prescribed worrisome narcotic drugs. They also visit quacks and practitioners of alternative medicine. In their extreme versions—multiple personalities, bizarre reports of rapes and satanic rituals—hysterics also seek publicity, either by way of the media or through the courts.

Many family doctors treat fibromyalgia, a modern version of what used to be called conversion hysteria. Some of these doctors have told me straightforwardly that this group of difficult patients is identical to the cluster of hysterical patients that Freud worked with early in his career. (Some colleagues are infuriated when I say there's nothing biologically wrong with patients who complain of fibromyalgia. I respond, by now wearily, saying, "Where's the evidence?")

These arguments illustrate why women were once called hysterics and why all attempts to consistently discover hysteria in men have failed: our culture and almost all other cultures demand that the strong-male archetype/stereotype is to be preserved. If women are hysterical and go to psychiatrists, it signals that, according to cultural habit, women can be thought of as needy, dependent, and on the scale of strength, inferior to men. The giddy woman who squeals at the sight of a mouse or a bug needs help, we say. If men are to look strong and potent, it follows that women, especially very womanly women, be given reduced stature—sickness. Men, on the other hand, prove their strength by choosing to visit psychiatrists far less often than women. To preserve men's precious image as Tarzan-of-the-Apes heroes, their habits are not judged as weak or silly. When masculine behaviour goes awry, it is judged to be a moral failure. For better or worse, the archetypal man is to be seen as robust and hearty—rough, competitive, rational. No illness or treatment for him.

These observations are wonderfully illustrated in a short story by Julian Barnes, "The Things You Know."[4]

To summarize, women/hysterics have pains, fears, the screaming meemies, and conversion symptoms. They are unwell and need treatment. Men/villains have moral failings, rape, bully, speed their cars, are rough competitors. They break rules and need discipline.

IN OUR CULTURE and in every culture, the thoughtful woman, the woman of sophisticated intelligence, is important, a stable influence on action-oriented men. She is the weaver who holds things together, who stands for life and survival. It's vitally important, says my thought experiment, that both the strong man (the action figure), and the strong woman (the wisdom figure), be familiar icons, the symbolic guarantors of two ways of life. The male icon creates safety; the woman icon creates *mêtis*, the wisdom Zeus got from his first wife. I could speculate about why these qualities are divided up the way they are, but in keeping with my determination to stay descriptive, I won't (truthfully, I don't speculate further because I have no answers to the questions that are being stirred up). This system is to my taste, as it is to anyone who has ever enjoyed an action film or appreciated the difference between a linebacker and a cheerleader.

Obviously, this paradigm, this configuration, this archetype, isn't an absolute: it's an image that orients us, keeps us from straying too far from what currently seems to work. Because it's not an absolute, it allows for a man to be a househusband, for a woman to be a professional boxer, and for people of either gender to be gay. But the jokes we make about househusbands and women boxers (behind closed doors, we make jokes about gays, too) reveal that we find less common role enactments quirky. Traditional role expectations are a reminder, powerfully insistent messages in all cultures. But it's important to remember that they're only messages. I don't worry about whether this is cultural or Darwinian; for me it's enough to say this is the way things are. Besides, there's no way to tease apart the relative contribution of

---

4 Julian Barnes, "The Things You Know," in *The Lemon Table* (New York: Alfred A. Knopf, 2004).

culture and genes. What's important is what people actually do; it's also important to keep in mind that these messages are so widespread that they seem to have value, even though I want to say it's not a moral issue. Since people of both sexes are fabulous and, I remind you, since people of both sexes are also jerks, to argue that these patterns are either good or bad strikes me as ridiculous (it's also, by the way, a pain in the neck to be a man and, equally, a pain in the neck to be a woman). Apart from using these observations to improve her thinking, an improvement that makes her better at helping her unhappy patients, the psychiatrist is only bemused by all this.

Be she angel, bitch, or fictional, without a man, no woman is a woman. The man does his duty by reminding the woman that wisdom isn't everything, that the rape metaphor, understood properly, guarantees the safety of the tribe, often showing itself as a wholesome moral will. The man accentuates this by pounding his fist on the table and being decisive about which television program will be watched, underlined by his taking top position in the bedroom. When the man dies, the woman is also dead, commits *sati* by mounting the funeral pyre with him.

It's said that no man is an island, and, be he real, symbolic, or rejected, without a woman, no man is a man. Whether he wants it or not, it is a woman's duty to remind him that restraint and thoughtfulness are vital. Once Siegfried and Brünnhilde have spent a night of love together, he realizes that from now on he is only an extension of her, her "arm." This explains why Eve was created from Adam's rib (the birth of male-type problem solving) and why Eve persuaded Adam to bite the apple of knowledge (the birth of female-type mystery and reinvention). Fortunately, the ways in which these archetypal actions are performed are not cast in stone; riffs and contrapuntal variations are the rule. It's no different in the gay world: although riffs and counterpoint may obscure what's going on, close attention makes it clear that manhood moments and womanhood moments are also alive and well there too.

When the psychiatrist is a man and the patient a woman, the powerful doctor-and-debilitated-patient configuration (a configuration that defines the patient as less well than the psychiatrist) makes its appearance according to well-known cultural archetypes. Commonest is that the male doctor is seen as the heroic dispenser of treatments and wisdom, the patient the grateful recipient of his services, although less commonly the psychiatrist is seen as harsh and vain. This includes the idea that in our culture and in every culture, the symbolic "alpha male" role is alive and well—the fighting hero who enforces moral codes, insists that children do their duty, ensures that the safety and honour of the tribe and of the nation survive. It's vitally important that the strong male be set up as a cultural institution, and concern about weak men is the guarantee that men will try to live up to that expectation. If the male doctor is not masculine but a wimp, so to speak, he will be gentle and delicately persuasive, which will be infuriating to some women patients, welcomed by others, and found to be ineffectual by still others. The male doctor may also perform his job in the language of the Lothario, the know-it-all, or the cynic, styles welcomed by some women, terrifying to others, seen as a time for counterattack by yet others.

When the doctor is a woman and the patient a man, things play out differently. The configurations are less well known to me, so I have to speculate. Will it be something we already know, a common interpersonal alignment: Maternal/grateful? Vamp/supplicant? Iron lady/subject? Will the woman psychiatrist dance flamenco, stamp out her space—"My space! My space!"—arrogant, scornful, daring her patient, "Are you man enough?" There's one thing I know with certainty: whether the psychiatrist is a man or a woman, the talking cure won't work the way I want it to work if the doctor thinks only of herself and portrays herself as the possessor of power and competence, and in synchrony, if the patient thinks only of himself and portrays himself as fragile and incapacitated.

Woman doctor/woman patient? Are the claws out? Will they be sisterly? Best friends? Share gossipy secrets? Instead of talking bullshit like men, will they talk intelligently? A psychiatric resident I'm working with, a woman, is good-looking and intelligent. As it turns out, her patient is also good-looking and intelligent. In their meetings, when they look at each other, I imagine them seeing a mirror image, charmed by each other's beauty and intelligence. Will this last forever? Simultaneously, I expect that eventually the claws will be out, and in the long run I may turn out to be right. Or wrong.

Gay psychiatrists will have to figure things out on a case-by-case basis (it's always case by case, anyway). Obviously, it partly depends on who at any particular moment claims the active role and who claims the passive (the contrasting roles of erastes and eromenos, the lover and the beloved) and whether power and control alternate or are divided up. Out of my sight, gay men tap into psychiatric talk, creative art, and creative sex more naturally than I do; I even suspect they have easier access than I to the eccentric thinking so necessary for the psychiatrist to do her work. For example: gay men, including gay psychiatrists, are interested in—and have fun with—camp. Camp is an excellent gizmo for the psychiatrist's tool chest, not buying into traditional truths about morality and aesthetics. The imaginative psychiatrist can therefore prod her patient to think about why he doesn't celebrate Liberace as enthusiastically as he celebrates Franz Liszt, doesn't put *The Sound of Music* in the same league as *Citizen Kane*, or doesn't applaud as loudly when the drag queen appears on stage as when Renée Fleming sings her aria.

About gay women psychiatrists, I also know little. But Janice Hannah, a gay woman psychiatrist I supervised, did give me a gift at the end of our year of working together, a bag of candies called black balls. I thanked her enthusiastically and explained that these candies are now hard to find, that as a child they had been my favourite candies (two for one cent). I went on at length about this. When I'd finished my rant, Dr. Hannah chuckled. "Look again," she said. When I looked, this time more closely, I saw that the black balls were—blue.

IN HIS SHORT story "A Painful Case," James Joyce says, "Love between man and man is impossible because there must not be sexual intercourse, and friendship between man and woman is impossible because there must be sexual intercourse," a comment that reminds me of my students, the psychiatric residents. It's easy for me to supervise male students; they know that love between a man and a man is impossible and that rivalry is the order of the day—and they'd best be careful with a teacher who will eventually give them a mark. They don't exactly say, "Yes, yes" and "Whatever you say," but when compared with women residents, an obedient attitude is in the air. Rarely will a male student argue, and when he does, he's likely to overdo it. Women don't bother with such nonsense; they know that between a man and a woman, there must be sexual intercourse, so rivalry is a lesser issue; they are confident. No matter how pedagogical and teacher-ish I aim to be, background archetypes are alive and kicking: with a man, I'm the dominant male and he has to be careful; with a woman, we are equals. Put two men together and the air will vibrate differently from when a man and a woman are put together. There's a pattern when women are put together, too, but about that, I'm less qualified to comment. But I am qualified to say that gender informs everything we do, and that includes doctor-patient relationships in one configuration or another. For example, when a woman works with a woman, they will, I suspect, talk more intimately with each other than do men. Men talk about sports, politics, and bullshit. They "brag" about sexual conquests, but it's mostly lies, almost never about women anyone else present knows, which is why I call it bullshit; I've never had a male friend say one word about his sexual relationship with his wife. Because men tend not to do this, I was shocked when as a young psychiatrist I began hearing from women patients that they discussed details of their marital sex life and other worries with sisters and close friends. An exception: one male friend did say to me of his wife, "If you're married to Helen, you have to be a necrophiliac," a humorous comment that is also a male vulgarity.

THAT I'M SEXUALLY straight, have standard romantic fantasies, and work hard at the expense of good fun means that despite what I'd like to think, I may not be a natural at the psychiatry business. What matters is that, despite portrayals—portrayals because all the world's a stage—of power or weakness or anything else, the psychiatrist is never to take a patient's self-depictions at face value. Rather, the psychiatrist is curious about how she and her patient are experimenting with their version of the game of life, and she never stops scratching her head about why this is the game they've together decided to play.

It's said that times have changed, but I suspect that in the past women both submitted ("Eek, eek!") and woke up ("Oops, did I just do that?"), just as in the present women both submit and wake up. It's tempting to believe that we think more clearly about psychiatrists and patients now, but I doubt this is true. Although we talk differently, we still have rules about how women and men are to act, and the difference we see in the year 2016 is only cosmetically different—we still recognize sexy women and sexy men and their identifying markers, including the markers called *submit* and *wake up* in women, and the markers called *wimp* and *bully-boy* in men.

PSYCHIATRIC CONFORMISTS WHO believe they know the causes of human oddity and human distress forget that, because we are not scientists, we psychiatrists can never have final answers. Like Mr. Casaubon in *Middlemarch*, the conformists want to believe there may, after all, be a key to all mythologies, that there'll soon be a long-dreamed-of breakthrough. Most psychiatric judgments, based as they are on mortal opinion, are tricky, but when the psychiatrist is faced with tricky misdemeanours, everything changes. No longer watchful and cautious, the psychiatrist speaks honestly, scolds, denounces, and penalizes. If a woman patient invites me to lunch, I think and invite her to think; if she tries to kiss me, I avoid the kiss, think, and invite her to think; if she grabs my crotch, I think and invite her to think, but I also push her away—politely—and ask a question: "What a bizarre thing to do. Why the devil would you do that? Obviously you're thinking about sex, but to touch me that way doesn't exactly strike me as sexual; it's more like wanting me to think ill of you." If the patient removes her clothes, it's assault, and I ought to call the police. I say "ought to," because really I don't know what I'd do.

And there is always a parallel story about the actions of sexually pushy male patients.

I'm making the argument that there is no tying such things together, no getting things clear, that there is no resting point, no foundation for things, that everything we humans do is arbitrary and therefore disconnected. I'd be contradicting my main argument if I tried to tie things together. It's what so many psychiatrists are doing: inventing a foundation for psychiatry that does not exist. There's no final answer for human behaviour without making an act of faith, and faith isn't my game. I don't care if people have faith in God, in BMWs, in opera, or in liberalism, as long as they 1) know it is a faith, and 2) don't impose it on anyone else. Religious people who speak of "faith" are admitting the truth, therefore doing the right thing, although they don't get much credit for this.

17

Los Expulsados and the Heroes

Busy remaking the world, man forgot to remake himself.

ANDREI PLATONOV,
Soviet existentialist author (1899–1951)

THE MAYAN RESIDENTS of San Juan Chamula, a town near San Cristóbal de las Casas, are determined to preserve their traditions. Tourists come to see the local customs, including culturally unique healing practices that one can watch in a building that once was a Roman Catholic church, a place analogous to the outpatient clinic in the hospital where I work. As in any good clinic, the Mayan practitioners see every troubled person who comes their way, both those with long-standing ailments and those whose problems are an emergency. There are many shamans conducting cures and exorcisms in the building, always surrounded by candles on the marble floor, bottles of Coca-Cola, and bottles of firewater. Since I'm a shaman myself, I paid close attention.

I was also here twenty years ago, when the main feature of the cure was the exorcism of a demon or a curse by transferring it to a chicken, which, at the end of the ritual, had its neck wrung. Miguel, my most recent guide on December 30, 2013, said the chicken ritual had become uncommon. Although I did find two chickens among the many shamans and clients, now firewater (called *pox*) was clearly the staple medium of the cure (it tasted like vodka). Miguel informed me that Coca-Cola, because it is gassy, induces the patient to burp out evil spirits—although later someone outside the building told me this theory was suspect, that my guide was entertaining me. The shaman I watched most closely took a mouthful of the firewater and, through pursed lips, blew a cloudy spray over the back of her sick patient's head and neck. There was also a lot of talking, chanting, and kneeling—and a few thumps on the back.

Later, Miguel told me the shaman's explanation of what had happened: the patient had been in a car accident a few months before, and although he'd suffered no injury, couldn't stop having bad dreams. "In Toronto this is called post-traumatic stress disorder," I told Miguel. I had to explain to him what this meant, and once he understood, he didn't approve. Rather than trauma, to him and the shaman the auspicious things were the *timing* of the accident and its *location*; these were the definitive causes of the patient's troubling dreams. Neither in Toronto nor in San Juan Chamula was it in fashion to speak about the patient's reaction to the accident being a mystery, a response unique to him or a message he wanted to convey, an opportunity to occupy the sick role briefly—or forever. And although I'm a Canadian through and through, I don't find these rituals as strange as you may think. These shamans are like me: confident, determined, and patient, sure they are on track in dealing with the problem of change. The shaman is a psychiatrist clone; she thinks she has the answer, just as I once did.

I'm so enamoured of these shamans that I have to remind myself they are not exclusively benign heroes; they are also a wolf pack. Woe betide a resident of San Juan Chamula who practises unfamiliar rituals, rituals other than those traditional in the town. Lest alien habits—mostly Christianity—infect and contaminate the local culture, the elders of the town expel deviants, including those who practise incorrect healing rituals—just as I, lest I infect and contaminate my own local culture, can be expelled if I don't practise "consensus medicine." Once expelled, dissident Mayans go to San Cristóbal de las Casas, where they are known as *los expulsados*. It's the identical fate suffered by psychiatric patients, especially those who are overtly crazy or weird, except that, instead of being banished to San Cristóbal, they are banished to a hospital or institution.

IN THE INDIGENOUS community of Lansdowne House in northern Ontario (population three hundred, accessible only in pontoon-equipped planes, now mostly abandoned by its inhabitants because the lawlessness and alcoholism had become intolerable), I've seen many examples of thinking that differs from the Canadian standard. One day in the middle of winter in Lansdowne House, a snowmobile was backed out of its shed and a passerby killed. The solution was to cut a hole in the ice on the lake and to dump the snowmobile into the hole. When I talked this over with some of the residents of Lansdowne House, I explained that in the south (southern Ontario, that is), if a driver kills a pedestrian, he may be held responsible for the death. My audience comprised phlegmatic indigenous people, who chuckled.

A native woman spoke to me on the path leading from Lansdowne House to the dock. This was unusual because the indigenous people in the town rarely talked to me, the visiting psychiatrist, on their own initiative (but they eagerly went to the nursing station when ophthalmologists visited because they brought with them boxes of eyeglasses). The woman was worried, she said, because she was jealous when her husband ran around with other women. Some discussion ensued, and eventually I understood that this made her feel different because other women in the community didn't become jealous. More discussion. Finally it became clear: she'd watched Hollywood films in the church on Sunday evenings and had learned two important things: first, white women in the movies are jealous when their husbands run around; second, white people talk to psychiatrists. Since one of her grandparents was white, she told me, she was jealous like a white woman and talked to a psychiatrist like a white woman.

SARITA WAS A young Indo-Canadian woman who had once been my secretary and who was a university student in India when I visited. She was a devotee of an Indian guru and had arranged for me to visit the ashram where he presided. When I landed in Delhi at 1:30 a.m., the guru's messenger Ananth met me. Ananth spoke English, one of the few on the ashram who did. The guru, Kripalu Maharaj, spoke no English. We headed southeast from Delhi by train to a tiny village near Kunda in Uttar Pradesh, a twelve-hour trip. On the last leg of our trip, a short hop by bus, I asked Ananth how to greet the Maharaji (the affectionate nickname used by devotees and the name I used for him). "Just do what I do," he answered.

The ashram was in a village, the residents of which were part of the guru's flock. At birth, they were assigned a destiny that excluded them from the formal ashram activities. Their karma, different from that of the devotees, was to be labourers and farmers. The ashram itself was made up of a cluster of dormitories and apartments and a meeting hall, where a party was going on when I arrived.

The party celebrated the Maharaji; he was an in-your-face hero, the star, the saviour. He sat on a platform—to me, it looked like a bed sprinkled with petals—and ate tidbits, some of which he tossed to the devotees crowded around. In two corners of the room were thrones, really heaps of colourful elevated pillows with gilded streamers and edging. I noticed spotlights and strategically placed video cameras pointed toward the thrones. Every eye was on the guru. The devotees cheerfully bounced him up and down. Although it was a party, only the guru was partying; the others cheered and applauded as he partied. He was brightly dressed with garlands around his neck and a large turban on his head (only for the party, I learned), and shoes with curled-up pointy toes. As he nibbled and shared his sweetmeats, the people threw flowers and petals. I was struck by his stature; even seated, he was clearly the tallest man in the room, over six feet, broad shouldered and strongly muscled. Although he was over seventy, his thick shoulders were particularly noticeable, shown off by sleeveless robes. He was clean-shaven and handsome, his features strong and bony.

I could see right away that the Maharaji's followers wished to make themselves—their souls—utterly subservient to him. Later, the devotees' thorough denial of their own interests—really a denial of their existence—became clearer. Always trying to discover the rituals people use to cure themselves, I suddenly grasped that their self-cure was to have no soul at all but to shadow, ape, and adapt themselves to the contrasting soul of the guru, which was alive, vivacious, throbbing.

The party was ending as Ananth and I arrived, and shortly after, some of his followers helped the guru down from his platform bed. Ananth was clearly sorry he'd missed the fun, and he took me to the side of the room where the Maharaji was removing his turban and some of the garlands. Ananth threw himself to the floor and kissed the maharaja's feet. "Just do what I do," he'd said to me on the bus. I also threw myself at the guru's feet (no kissing though). When I stood, he made a joke, which was translated by Ananth. "'It's good you are here. I'm the one who needs a psychiatrist.'"

I made a joke back. "Maybe we are in the same business."

He'd sized me up and instantly realized I was no devotee. The people surrounding us looked puzzled, probably because visitors were usually awed and submissive, and my polite conversation probably looked irreverent.

During my time on the ashram, the Maharaji didn't pester me as he did the others. He nagged his devotees to take notes when he lectured, to have their books with them, sometimes to come forward and dance. From the luxury of his thrones, he lectured twice a day, every word and gesture recorded by two cameras, later to be made into DVDs for sale in the business office. When he and I passed each other, he would acknowledge me politely.

Each day started at 4:00 a.m. with an insistent blast from a ram's horn; continuous chanting began and didn't stop until 11:00 p.m. In the morning, everyone gathered in the meeting hall for prayer and meditation, although the Maharaji didn't appear until later in the day. Most were Indians, although some had once been Indian immigrants in Canada and the United States. A white Australian woman who'd had a bookstore in Sydney before moving to the ashram told me she'd been looking for a guru for many years, and when she met the Maharaji, she knew this was the ashram for her. An American man, also white, was clearly a madman. He stood in one position for many hours a day and rarely spoke.

Several women spent the day cooking. Three times a day we lined up with our tin plates and were served the same bland food as was served at the cult's two branches in Toronto: cauliflower, lentils, naan, yogurt. There were no spices or meat and, as I remember it, nothing green. We ate with our hands, sitting on the dusty ground, a row of men on one side, women on the other. In the meeting hall men and women also sat separately.

Often, right after the guru's lecture, one of his assistants—there were several on the ashram, all referred to as "Didi" and dressed in identical orange saris—translated for three or four of us who spoke only English. At the translation session, the ideas seemed silly, repetitive claims of peace and eternal wisdom for those who listened carefully to the guru's message. Because I asked questions, I caught Didi's attention and she invited me to the guru's garden to discuss these philosophical matters in more detail. I watched her closely. She was from Tahiti, a very beautiful young woman, golden brown and tender-looking. Lusciously, her skin looked too tight for her body. At close quarters I noticed that her face was shining with happiness, that she was in a state of ecstasy. *She is so aroused*, I imagined, *that here in the guru's garden, I could seduce her, and she would barely realize what I was up to. She'd think she was making love with the guru or with someone assigned by the guru to make love with her.*

Didi explained that the Maharaji kept spiritual and physical things apart; he tried not to treat physical ailments himself. But it was known on the ashram that he sometimes came to devotees in their dreams and healed their ailments. It was unheard of to ask the guru for healing, because help came by grace. Occasionally he cured people directly, usually by looking at the affliction fleetingly, by touching the body part, or by saying the name of the affliction or of the body part that was affected. Mostly, his cures were carried out secretly—secret even to the person healed.

The guru lived on behalf of his devotees. He partied, feasted, had a sex life—he was married—and had children. The devotees lived vicariously. I once watched the Maharaji go into a trance, peace and bliss in his face. And then, to my amazement, he had or mimed having an orgasm—heavy breathing, glowing perspiration, pelvic thrusting. A few months later I told my thoughts about the orgasm to another devotee who lived in Toronto. "He was having an orgasm or pretending to have an orgasm. Do you devotees not see that?"

"Well, of course he was having an orgasm," she answered. "We live through him and he has to have orgasms on our behalf. Christianity is so impractical."

The Maharaji was the cure. The devotees gave up their souls and were reborn in him, like those reborn in Christ. But the devotees did it with a vengeance. In Canada, those who were serious about their faith knew when the Maharaji had his daily bowel movement; they had theirs at the same time. He ate; they, thousands of kilometres and nine-and-a-half time zones away, ate. He prayed; they prayed. Every few days he visited his garden and the devotees were allowed to take pictures. He smirked as many kneeled at his feet and kissed his hands. Perhaps "smirked" is too mild; I got the sense that he found the devotees to be ridiculous and that he scorned them.

The devotees were examples of the cure by rebirth of the soul—but in this instance, reborn in their leader, not in themselves. Although he was a real devotee, Ananth didn't seem as awestruck and dazzled by the Maharaji as did the others on the ashram. He and I chatted about secular things; no one else did that. He liked my T-shirts and I liked his Indian dhotis, so we traded.

A month after my trip to the ashram, a parcel arrived from Kripalu Maharaj—from his business office, I assumed. It contained a scarf, a photo of the soles of the guru's feet (it's now on my fridge), and sticks of incense. Then, *six* months after my trip to the ashram, I received something different, something worrisome: a letter from Sarita, my one-time secretary. She was on the ashram without money and could not leave. Her mother had control of Sarita's money in Toronto, and because her mother was also a devotee and went along with the guru's wishes, she was a prisoner. Kripalu Maharaj had reassured her that he had a splendid career in mind for her, that he planned to send her to Harvard Business School. She would then become the manager of his ashrams, multi-million-dollar enterprises that were (and still are) among the largest in India. I sent Sarita a plane ticket and some cash, and she returned to Canada. Then, twenty *years* after my trip to the ashram, I had an email from a woman in Texas. She'd been a devotee for fifteen years and had read what I'd said about the guru in another book, and she informed me that my suspicions about him were correct. She herself had written a book about her experiences as a devotee for fifteen years.[1] The guru's ashrams, both in India and in the US, were replete with sexual corruption. He'd been charged with rape both in India and in Trinidad. Kripalu Maharaj died before the courts had finished their work.

1 Karen Jonson, *Sex, Lies, and Two Hindu Gurus: How I Was Conned by a Dangerous Cult—and Why I Will Not Keep Their Secrets* (Austin, Texas: Rishika Books, 2012).

THE IMPORTANCE OF leadership figures cannot be overestimated: John F. Kennedy, Adolf Hitler, Pierre Trudeau, Chairman Mao, Jesus of Nazareth, Napoleon Bonaparte, Kongzi (Confucius), Winston Churchill, and once upon a time, a series of psychiatric stars—Sigmund Freud, Carl Jung, Erich Fromm, as well as the one I worked under, Karl Menninger—who were incarnations of the hero archetype. All these leaders are men, of course, but why the archetypal array is so commonly set up that way, I don't know. (Nor do I know why fictional monsters in the funnies are men, whereas in ancient Greece monsters were often women. To add to the inconsistency, in south-east Asia female dancers are beautiful and delicate, whereas male dancers wear false faces, the ugly grimacing faces of demons or dogs.) Examined closely, many of the heroes I've identified turn out to have been worthy leaders tainted by personal foibles; others were just plain evil. But millions adored them despite their foibles and badness, just as we admire and think well of our doctors, despite foibles and worse. I'd estimate that three quarters of patients think their psychiatric doctor is wonderful; a quarter of them think the opposite, that their doctor is ordinary or stupid.

As they should, doctors exploit this idealization, using it to comfort sick people. The doctor's imagined authority position gets many patients through difficult times, especially on the frequent occasions when there is nothing substantial that needs to be done or can be done. Until 150 years ago, a doctor's primary role was to act as a supervisor of what was going on, a spectator who gave comfort as diseases ran their natural course. Dr. Behrens, the tuberculosis specialist who directed the sanatorium in Thomas Mann's *The Magic Mountain*, had an array of dramatic treatments at hand, and as we now know, all were useless if not harmful; I doubt that rest cures, high altitude, enormous nourishing meals, artificial pneumothoraces, and rib resections did any good. I'm sorry to disappoint my readers, but psychiatry is little different, except that, in addition to having no real treatments, we also are responsible for the treatment of no real diseases.

As distinct from psychiatry, technological medicine now has real and effective treatments for many diseases. Nevertheless, the power of the doctor's comforting role cannot be overemphasized, and at times this causes trouble, particularly for the psychiatrist. When the psychiatrist has in mind serious personal change for her patient, she aims to tease apart everything the patient says—including analyzing the nature and occasions of the patient's idealizations of her and, less easy to get at, her patient's dislike or contempt for her. With psychiatrists, such idealizations are almost always present because the quarter of patients who are indifferent or who dislike their psychiatric doctor will often have dropped out. In the clinic and the hospital this isn't a problem because the psychiatrist straightforwardly exploits such idealizations to get people through a rough patch. But if her aim is a change in the way her patient lives his life, she doesn't exploit the patient's idealizations; instead she studies what's going on and carefully and consistently analyzes it. Kripalu Maharaj, one of the more monstrous leaders, *used* the devotee's idealizations for his own evil ends.

KARL MENNINGER'S BOOKS convinced me I should train in his program. Dr. Karl, a tall, enthusiastic man with a broad smile, was a show-business character and a genius. His passion for social causes immunized me against those who feel psychiatry should be scientific and technological. I first met him at a gathering of new psychiatric residents. "I'm Karl Menninger," he said, with a Kansas twang (to this Canadian, the twang was exotic). He wore a suit with a chequered shirt—to me a "cowboy" shirt—and string tie. He immediately introduced me to each member of the group with whom he had been chatting, people who I quickly realized were other new residents whose names Karl Menninger had just learned. He never forgot my name either.

Dr. Karl's passion for social causes had a strong effect on us. For example, he said that to call someone schizophrenic was no different from calling someone a nigger. For many years, I struggled with that notion—it seemed too harsh and I feared that if I adopted it, I would be seen as a fool. Now I know I hesitated only because of my cowardice, fear of going against the profession's sacred beliefs. Karl Menninger could say it, but I couldn't. His chief campaign was against all psychiatric diagnosis, which to him was just psychiatric name calling. He also raged against the killing of fur-bearing animals, bad prison conditions, and the mistreatment of North American indigenous people. These passions made passion legitimate and inspired me to adopt passions of my own.

I tried to identify with Karl Menninger's way of thinking, but identifying deeply means changing your soul, and such things are hard to achieve by merely trying. A rock-solid identification with someone means *becoming* him, *being* him, a fundamental reorientation that, despite its profundity, is done unwittingly. Instead of admiring and loving Dr. Karl, basking for a while in my hero worship, I complained about his showiness, his carelessness about detail, and his tolerance of the sycophants who fluttered around him. I grabbed onto his virtues and claimed them as my own. Rarely acknowledging that he had inspired me, I decided early on that I would be a psychiatric idealist: I'd never waver from my duty, never make jokes about patients, and never, ever think of patients as having a status less worthy than mine. Karl Menninger didn't say most of these things explicitly, but he exuded those attitudes, and though I didn't see it at the time, his attitudes fell on fertile ground.

His image stood on the shoulders of the other, earlier models I had tried out: my high school principal Norman McLeod, for example, whom I admired and, using a clever form of split thinking, whom I thought I scorned. He suggested that instead of saying, "Jill read a book *while* Jack ran up the hill," I could say, "... *whereas* Jack ran up the hill." There was also my Uncle Charlie, the swimming teacher with muscles, and Dr. Broad, our family doctor who, knowing that as enemy aliens we had no money, had charged us no fees during World War II. I'd picked up the scent of idealism before I met Dr. Karl, but without receiving credit for it at the time, he gave me a language for it and a cause. No psychiatric name calling, never abandon hope for anyone—*anyone*—and offer help to all who ask, no matter how stupid or hopeless they *appear* to be.

At eighty-three, my hunt for a hero isn't over, but the one I loved most—even though I didn't know I loved him when I was his student—was Karl Menninger. At the time, it was all about figuring out how to turn myself into a psychiatrist—a real psychiatrist, not one who chased symptoms away as quickly as possible—and watching the role take ever-deeper possession of me.

Karl Menninger knew he was a public figure. Some saw his behaviour as a product of too much ego, but I now know better. This was no cheap vanity, but the sign that he was a creature of life, a warrior, a psychiatric Muhammad Ali. He was never a thin-blooded obsessive, and his flamboyance woke us up and made us think. Karl Menninger was enacting his destiny, a social role that owned him, body and soul. Drama attracts attention and Dr. Karl attracted it wherever he went. I took him to lunch in Toronto many years later and, although he didn't speak in a loud voice, others in the restaurant noticed him; when he went to the washroom, a person at the next table leaned over and asked, "Who *is* that?" He had presence.

Each Sunday Dr. Karl taught a bible study class at the hospital. The patients in the C.F. Menninger Hospital couldn't figure this out. Some thought he must be nuts; others suspected he was a Christian missionary. They must have been surprised when his subversive mind—not sacrilegious, subversive—stirred them up. What in the world could be going on when the most famous psychiatrist in the world teaches bible studies? The psychiatric community shared their confusion. "He's nuts." "It's show biz." "Dr. Karl is just doing his number again."

During the first year of our training we could invite Dr. Karl to consult with our hospital units, so I arranged for him to come to our little team meeting. The five of us had to wait six months, but he eventually came. On the big day, Dr. Karl arrived with a photographer, a dog, and a dog handler. Our reactions were mixed. Was this a special day? Was he a fool? A hero? A god? Never underestimate the importance of drama. After such an entrance, who could forget what happened later?

I presented a case of chronic depression, a woman who lived several hundred kilometres away in western Kansas. When she arrived to be interviewed, there was more show business. When the woman was seated, Dr. Karl looked at her with a puzzled expression on his face. Suddenly he stood. "Sarah," he said, "what are you doing here?" We were stunned; patients are *never* to be addressed informally, by their first names. Sarah also rose, they embraced, and both burst into tears. It turned out they had attended high school together fifty years earlier.

And what did Dr. Karl recommend? It all seems impossibly silly today, but he recommended that she fly to Topeka three times a week to meet with a psychoanalyst. She was wealthy, so this posed no financial problems. To make such a recommendation with the sparse information he had seemed outrageous, but don't forget Dr. Karl was a dramatist and a teacher. He was telling Sarah there was hope for her, that help was available, and he taught us youngsters the same lesson.

On Saturday mornings, Dr. Karl held a colloquium. Most of the psychiatrists and students attended, perhaps a hundred people in all. On picnic tables around the perimeter of the room were duplicated copies of articles and book chapters the great man had read during the preceding week and that he thought would be of interest. The colloquium consisted of Karl Menninger's commentary on the articles that had stirred his thinking.

In the front row sat senior colleagues, who acted as intellectual consultants. Most were psychiatrists and psychologists, but often there was an English or philosophy professor as well. If he got stuck in his thinking—he often forgot words or phrases, a tic that kept the audience on edge—he would turn to his front row and say, "Harold, what is it that Shakespeare [Erasmus, Freud] said about this? What was that quote?" And the colloquium was always spiced with complaints about social problems such as crime and jail conditions.

"Uh, how many of you have visited the Shawnee County jail?" he asked one Saturday morning. "It's just up the street here. It's a good jail, mostly because of the work of one woman, a wise woman who lives here in our town. As responsible citizens, have you visited it?"

The audience was silent and a few people raised their hands.

"Well, if y'all haven't visited our local jail, are you any different from the Germans, who, after World War II, claimed no knowledge of concentration camps?" What else could one hope for from a teacher? He made us think. Having chastised us, Dr. Karl proceeded to rub it in.

"I tried to get some prisoners to come to the colloquium today, but nobody seemed able to authorize it. But I phoned the state penitentiary and they agreed to let the Leavenworth State Prison choir come to meet with y'all." Sure enough, at that very moment, the choir entered through the rear doors. They were in chains and, within minutes, the audience was in tears. Naturally enough, melodrama was compounded by more melodrama: they sang "Nobody Knows the Trouble I've Seen." As flair ruled Dr. Karl's soul, he upset us by polling the prisoners. We all knew the questions and what the answers would be.

A black prisoner. "What was your offence, sir?"

"Break and enter."

"What is your sentence?"

"Five years."

A white prisoner. "What was your offence, sir?"

"Break and enter."

"What is your sentence?"

"Three years."

Murderers? A black man: twenty years; a white man: twelve years.

As I watched Dr. Karl's performance, I realized his theatricality wasn't a quirk. He was an icon, madly doing his duty and performing his role. The power of roles became clearer as I watched him. I saw how I enacted the complementary role of student. Karl Menninger was my one and only chance to be stamped into a psychiatrist.

What else did Karl Menninger do? Well, he rode a horse, and he made sure we saw him, dressed as a Kansas cowboy, riding the grounds of the Menninger Foundation. He was seventy years old. And each day, he read a book and wrote a review of it for publication (I think he'd made a New Year's resolution to do this for one year). I would see him at concerts, busily reading. Where he found the time, I don't know, but he also carried on an enormous correspondence. He once said that he wrote forty letters a day—not emails. He also lectured to the psychiatric residents every week, something unheard of for the director of such a large institution. Usually, the lecturing duties of directors and heads of departments of psychiatry elsewhere consist of ritual introductory remarks made at the beginning of the academic year.

In September 1961 we had our first psychiatric lecture in the auditorium of the Winter VA Hospital. Sure enough, Menninger appeared at the front of the room, wearing a professional white coat. In his hand, he had a list of the psychiatric residents. "Instead of starting at the beginning of the alphabet," he said, "let's start at the end today. Let's see. Dr. Warme? Is Dr. Warme here? Ah, there you are. Would you please come up to the front?" There were two chairs. "I have a patient for you. Please interview him for fifteen or twenty minutes, then let him go back to the ward. His name is Mr. Donaldson." Dr. Karl gave me no advice, no support, no encouragement.

The patient, a young man of about twenty-five, came in. I introduced myself and we shook hands. His handshake was feeble, and he sat silently during the whole so-called interview. I asked why he was in the hospital, what he needed help with, whether I could be of help or answer any questions. I offered him a cigarette, guessed out loud that he must be feeling uncomfortable, and reassured him about the forty people watching. He didn't say a word. In the end, I probably needed reassurance more than he did. I was humiliated and felt on the verge of a nervous breakdown. After fifteen minutes, I told Mr. Donaldson he could return to his ward.

"That was fine, Dr. Warme," Dr. Karl said before turning to the class and asking for their opinions. A number of suggestions were offered on how I might have proceeded and obtained a better result; other people discussed how I might have made Mr. Donaldson more comfortable.

Dr. Karl looked amused. "Well, Dr. Warme, let me now tell you something. Mr. Donaldson is actually not a patient. He is one of your colleagues, a fellow resident whom I asked to be the patient for today. I told him not to speak." I, for my part, was not amused. In fact, I hated him then for humiliating me.

Dr. Karl wanted to make the point that when interviewing patients, we already have the interpersonal skills that make for a worthwhile interview, that there is less to learn about interviewing than we sometimes think. To cling to an artificial "professional" style or to a predetermined series of questions is futile. He wanted to illustrate that when faced with an impasse, I had no recourse but to fall back on my personal methods. It was part of his message of humanism, dramatized at my expense. As I write these words, I wonder whether the interviewing seminar I later conducted for twenty years was born out of that first humiliation Dr. Karl had inflicted on me. Wasn't it true that my own interviews were always a dramatic illustration of my social ingenuity, and never demonstrations of a pre-established technique?

At the end of our first year of training, we were required to write a dissertation before moving on to the second year of the program. I was a conscientious student and the first of the residents to complete and turn in my paper. Two days later, it was sent back. Dr. Karl had written on it: "I've only read one sentence. It's a dreadful sentence and I refuse to read any further." I was both humiliated and frightened. Would I have to produce a new dissertation? Was I in trouble with the great man? Hopefully, I thought, he wouldn't remember who I was, and I wouldn't be in jeopardy. I couldn't believe that Karl Menninger himself took the trouble to read dissertations. There were hundreds of teachers around, and *he* read dissertations? In despair, I went to my supervisor.

He smiled. "Dr. Karl does this every year. Change the first sentence, change the title, and wait a few weeks before resubmitting it."

A few years after I left Kansas, I had an article published in a journal. Within a few days, a letter arrived, three sentences long.

> Dear Warme,
>
> I appreciated the nice article of yours in the current issue of the *American Journal of Psychiatry*. I didn't understand what you said about ethology.
>
> I trust things are going well for you and your family.
>
> Sincerely,
>
> Karl Menninger, MD

I was flattered the great man had written, since I had been one of hundreds of students. In a few weeks I wrote back, explaining what I had meant. Within days I had an answer. This pattern continued. Karl Menninger would answer my letters immediately, while I would answer after a few weeks. I didn't want to burden him, you see—he had to be very busy—but it turned out that he was *never* too busy. The correspondence petered out because of me. For Dr. Karl, it was his *duty* to write to me. It was his duty to be who he was, the American psychiatric culture hero. These days, such heroes are few and far between.

On another occasion, Dr. Karl was in Toronto and I took him on a tour of the city. As we drove by the Clarke Institute of Psychiatry where I worked, I shyly said to him, "Dr. Karl, now *I* am a teacher."

He harrumphed, saying, "This isn't the time to be a teacher, Warme. Now you have to do research."

Bastard, I thought. *Aren't you the one who taught me research has little to do with our work?* But then he spoke up again.

"I don't mean that silly research that measures statistics and surveys populations. I mean there ought to be research done on problems like epidemic greed and vengeance, problems that cause far more trouble than the so-called diseases everyone is so busy treating."

IF YOU'D BEEN invited, and if you didn't inform Florence that you wouldn't be coming to the seminar, you might never be invited again. She was tough like that, but it didn't matter because we all loved her, adored her. Why is it the purview of women to host "salons," lead reading groups, attract intellectuals? Florence Rosberg's group was definitely a salon, the members English professors, professional actors, and Florence's personal friends. I was the token psychoanalyst. We met irregularly, usually when Florence had a bright idea. She'd then inform one or more of us that we were to make a presentation, the format including a seminar leader (not her; she sat at the back and rarely spoke), a presentation, and formal discussions. Occasionally we'd read a play aloud, perhaps Shakespeare, and if lucky, I'd get to read the role of some minor character. Inspired by the actors, those plays were thrilling, even for those of us who were usually inarticulate.

I didn't know Florence when I first heard from her. She charmed me on the phone and I agreed to come to the next meeting. I knew it was my duty to speak up at the meeting—I suspect it was an audition—so I made a few "psychoanalytic" comments about what had been presented. I could not attend the next meeting but had a call from Florence a few days afterward. "I understand you're interested in Thomas Mann, and I'd love it if you'd pick one of his short stories for us and give us a discussion of it."

I demurred. "Gee, Florence, someone has misinformed you. I have a bit of an interest in TM, have read *Buddenbrooks* and *The Magic Mountain*, but I'm certainly no TM scholar."

"Come along and do it, darling. You can give us a psychoanalytic view of him. Just pick a short story. I know you'll do something terrific. Someone at the last seminar mentioned your interest in TM, and now the whole group is excited to hear your thoughts about him."

It would be impossible to reproduce the charm, the power, and flattery with which Florence said this. I don't know how she did it, but she'd implanted blatant insanity into me. Once she'd spoken, I knew three important things: she loved me more than anyone else in the world; I was obviously the most brilliant person on the planet; whatever I said about Thomas Mann at the seminar would be extraordinary.

I discussed Mann's short story "Tristan." And I learned something: a literary and a psychoanalytic commentary on a story are the same thing.

Every member of the seminar had the same reaction to Florence—she was our pushy, amazing, mother-heroine. As of this writing she has been dead for ten years, but when those of us who'd been part of the seminar meet, we immediately shake our heads in amazement as we reminisce. She was powerful, the tough version of empathy.

THESE REMARKABLE PEOPLE consume the same oxygen as psychiatrists. All have foibles, and some are scoundrels. All are tiles in the mosaic that makes up our world, players in the complicated maelstrom called human life. None are gods, just as no psychiatrists are gods.

18

An Experiment: Ward H

Don't ask me. Ask the nurses. The nurses are with him all the time. They know what's going on.

KARL MENNINGER

PSYCHIATRY IS ABOUT the elusive and the human, and it should be talked about using the same language we use when talking about movies and novels, about your neighbour's secret drug habit, and about how your cousin fell in love and married, then beat up his wife. That's it. Instead of meaningless diagnostic words, stick with what I call "ways of life."

Having concluded this, talking doctors like me are at risk of forgetting something obvious: only a fraction of the people we see are interested in philosophers like Wittgenstein and in linguistics, especially at first. Those who are find satisfaction in private offices on St. Clair Avenue West in Toronto, on Park Avenue in New York, or on Harley Street in London. There, the upper middle class find a niche that echoes their own way of life: soft lighting, good furniture, conversation with a business-suited professional.

Many patients are desperate, even suicidal, and go to emergency departments, while others are so crazy or disabled that they have to be in a protected environment—a hospital or, better, a foster home located in a neighbourhood.

Because they are run by doctors, I'm worried about modern asylums. I'm uneasy that we doctors have been spoiled by our first patients—the cadavers in our anatomy labs—and will always think the ideal patient should be passive, lie still, accept our dissections, and swallow the pills we give them. Not that I think any other group of people would do better; the babying of the mad, and the extreme opposite, the bullying of the mad, will go on forever. Warnings, reminders, scoldings, and strong laws will always be needed. I sometimes doubt that talking doctors should even visit psychiatric hospitals or act as consultants, and I dream that residents of asylums will some day visit doctors *outside of the asylum*, at a medical clinic or a private office. The medical model works well in a clinic, an emergency room, and a doctor's office, but what I see on psychiatric inpatient units isn't right. Staff members consistently fall into a trap, submitting to a flawed part of medical magic by embracing the hospital version of medicine that works very well for broken bones and leukemia but is counterproductive for psychiatric patients. In psychiatric hospitals, the subdue-people-with-drugs standard is universal.

Many psychiatric facilities, including the hospital where I work, know about this problem, and they are made to resemble the community at large. But a hospital shouldn't merely resemble communities. It should be broken into dozens of group homes in the outside world where other people live. But we doctors are in the habit of doing things for people, so I expect that, even if the hospital is integrated into a neighbourhood, our patients will still not have the thing they most need: responsibility. Even the idea of group homes may be too weak; perhaps psychiatric patients should be in their *own* homes, an extreme idea that imposes on their families endless heartaches and work. Rarely are patients so wildly bizarre or threatening that no matter where they are they must be physically restrained or given powerful drugs.

I recently spent a day with a psychiatrist who works in a clinic that is responsible for patients who are integrated into the community. Some live in subsidized apartments, others with relatives (the clinic gives a lot of support to the families), a few live in foster homes. The psychiatrist visits the patients twice a week. The visits I watched discouraged me. Most of the patients in subsidized apartments were doing nothing when we arrived; some sat on the edge of their beds, others on their couches, often with the television on. All were on powerful drugs, obvious at first glance because they acted spooky—as though pithed, in other words. When one patient said he was going to make an appointment with a dentist, the psychiatrist supported his status as being a person who has been pithed and said she would take care of setting up the appointment. Conversations with these patients were no different from conversations on inpatient units: subdued by antipsychotic medications, patients had little interest in talking. Except for one manic woman, the patients had been dehumanized by two things—drugs and lack of responsibility.

As opposed to my daydreams, *real* change will require painful soul-searching, a new medical/psychiatric world in which doctors de-emphasize their own role, passing on to other experts the real task, teaching patients how to find housing, earn and handle money, get a job, enjoy music/movies/art/games/exercise, horse around, garden, flirt, and use a chainsaw. If he is very crazy, the patient can still see a psychiatrist; at best, he himself will phone a doctor or a clinic to make an appointment. If he's too crazy to make a phone call, someone will help him, if necessary accompany him to the doctor's office or clinic. They won't do this out of superficial kindness and only if the patient truly cannot manage it on his own.

The patient's doctor, also caught in the medical tradition, will be tempted to act fast, give a subduing pill, or recommend a hospital. It's possible that doctors can be trained to do more than prescribe a pill, but I'm not sure it would work; doctors expect patients to comply with the prescribed treatments, exactly the assignment psychiatric patients don't need. In my ideal institution, the patient would also make his own dental appointments, go to church rather than being visited by a chaplain, and get a haircut somewhere in the neighbourhood. If I could figure out how to find a barber in chaotic Yangon in Myanmar even though no one spoke English (I gestured and said, "Buzz, buzz"), and even though most of the barbers waved me away because they feared I was a white demon, I'm sure a patient can get a haircut in Toronto. How do I know? Well, for example, if he's a smoker, even in chaotic Yangon and even if he's psychotic, he'll find a way to bum a cigarette—just as he'd do in a psychiatric hospital, where cigarettes are one of the most highly sought-after items. Extremely crazy people know how to find and get what they truly want, no matter what it is.

IN THE 1960S, Topeka State Hospital in Kansas carried out a project that attempted to avoid the problems of total institutions. It was designed and implemented by two psychologists, Nick Colarelli and Saul Siegel.[1] To demonstrate that a non-medical asylum system was possible, a women's ward, Ward H (originally it had been what in those days was called the Violent Ward), was designated to be completely operated by psychiatric aides. Doctors, psychologists, nurses, and social workers held no authority and gave no input into how things should be run. For legal purposes, Ward H technically had a doctor, and for one year I held that bureaucratically necessary position. I visited the ward three times a week for an hour, meeting only with the aides, and working at a full-time job elsewhere. Almost exclusively, the meetings were about the ward's goings-on, very gossipy, often fun, but they also included complaints and pessimism. As I came and went, I chatted with the patients informally but took part in no treatment initiatives or decisions. The ward was an odd place, some of the patients threatening, others bizarrely preoccupied by their own inner worlds, still others posturing or immobile, caught up in private reveries. Most were on antipsychotic drugs, and part of my assignment was to refresh prescriptions when necessary, changing dosages based on the advice of the psychiatric aides, the only people on the unit who were supposed to make treatment decisions.

The aides embraced their new role enthusiastically. In contrast to nurses and aides on traditional wards, they had little interest in the drugs given to their patients, only occasionally asking me to increase the dosage of a drug, more commonly asking me to reduce the amount prescribed or to discontinue the drugs completely. Although it took a few months, the aides developed methods of their own, methods outside

---

1 Details about this experiment can be found in Nick J. Colarelli and Saul M. Siegel, *Ward H: An Adventure in Innovation* (New York: D. Van Nostrand Co., 1966), and in Gordon Warme, "Consulting with Aide-Therapists," *Archives of General Psychiatry* Vol. 13 (November 1965): p. 432–38.

of the usual medical/psychiatric culture. They managed patients and made decisions with no reversion to disease and treatment language, instead staying with a language based on ordinary human practices, often those used in raising children. At first I liked the new language, although today I think of it as moralistic, just as crippling as the language of disease. They yelled at patients, scolded them, commanded them, and told them to shut up, but they also loved and kissed their patients, hugged them, teased them, and conspired with them. I, in turn, came to love the aides.

Some excluded their patients from the ward as punishment, locking the doors so they couldn't get in, but they also took patients on personal grocery-shopping trips, into their homes to have sleepovers, and to their children's birthday parties. They also brought their children to the ward. Inspired by them, I brought my two-month-old son to the ward for a visit. The patients looked closely at the baby, and those usually withdrawn and bizarre also stared out of the corner of their eyes, even though they tried not to let on.

One aide said, "Make your bed, you lazy nigger" (she was a "nigger" herself), but also brought her baby and her children to the ward. She once had a patient look after her baby while she did an errand off the ward (I'm not sure about this memory, but the image illustrates the flavour of what was going on).

In the home of one of the aides, I saw two patients acting as though they were part of the household. One helped with the cooking while the other sewed while sitting on the glider on the porch. (I can't remember why I would have been in the aide's home.)

No one reported this, but I know they hit their patients. I once came upon an aide spanking a patient who was flopped over her knee, so cartoonish that I couldn't tell whether it was a punishment or a joke. The patient was a voluptuously gorgeous woman, but her black skin was horribly disfigured because she'd once set her own hair on fire, and startling white scars covered her skull and one side of her face.

I DIDN'T UNDERSTAND then that the model of child-rearing is no better than the disease model; it didn't solve the problems of overprotectiveness, of the patients having no responsibility, and of *being treated as lesser citizens*. Like doctors and nurses on traditional psychiatric wards, the aides couldn't figure out how to treat a crazy person as an equal, and overprotectiveness was the order of the day. It didn't occur to the aides that the patients should take responsibility for themselves, wash their own clothes, clean the floors (cleaners did this), or visit their families (the aides were adamant that families had a bad effect on patients; they, the aides, felt *they* were the only decent "parents"). Most of us are like that. When we see a stubborn or rude child, we are quick to be judgmental, to think that the child had bad parenting. "I could do it better," we think. The only real advantage of a system like the Ward H project was that, without the expense of psychiatrists, psychologists, or social workers, it was cheaper to run.

The Ward H project lasted for several years and was deemed a great success, the patients considered "definitely" improved. I was in enthusiastic agreement. Now, forty-five years later, I'm skeptical—I doubt we were right. But even though no one was cured, the goodness of that world touched me—and all the people who knew about the project. It also stimulated me to think: *this is humanity at its best*. Now, I would add a rider: *it was also humanity not up to snuff*. I'll be direct and bold like the aides who worked on Ward H. Despite spankings, curses, and penalties—*because of* spankings, curses, and penalties—that is to say, because the aides did not think of their patients as biologically inferior specimens of humanity, *instead thought of them as morally inept and immature*, it was humanity at its best and, because life is contradictory, humanity not up to snuff.

19

Psychiatry Does Not Progress

When we are not sure, we are alive.

GRAHAM GREENE

THIS IS THE golden age of biological psychiatry; it's in its prime—and its ecstasy. I grew up during the previous golden age, that of psychoanalytic psychiatry and its ecstasy. Like the biological psychiatrists who now cure every psychiatric misery, we, equally filled with hysterical enthusiasm and just as convinced we were in our prime, also cured every psychiatric misery—or so we said. Both then and now, psychiatrists have believed in discoveries, that psychiatric illness is soon to be conquered. I'm sorry to say that, tragic for them and for those who love them, most of those who are fully mad are doomed to be extremely odd and to be social problems for the rest of their lives. I don't promote biological psychiatry (its empty rhetoric is everywhere), and I support psychoanalytic psychiatry (still the Holy Grail for some, an interesting talking experience for others) only cautiously because I've assigned myself another job. My new job is to remind everyone of something obvious, something that's unfamiliar to the public but that every psychiatrist knows: all indicators of psychiatric illness—including the delusions and hallucinations of the people said to have schizophrenia—are social practices. There are no abnormal chemicals and no psychoanalytic complexes or fixations in sight. Just as the psychologically oriented psychoanalysts once had a delirious belief in psychiatric progress, the biologists now have a delirious belief in "breakthroughs," more safely referred to as being "on the verge" of breakthroughs.

In other medical fields when a patient complains of symptoms, thinking about chemical and organ pathology has a practical payoff, not because there's a mysterious hidden world behind the symptoms but because when we look, we find actual physical or chemical abnormalities. But in psychiatry, we've looked and looked again, and there's no hint of anything to be found. If nothing is there, there's no payoff in acting as though there is. In all—yes, *all*—other medical fields, there *is* a payoff. For example, if a cough is considered to be a sign, it makes sense to look for something in the throat and lungs—a viral or bacterial infection, a cancer, a foreign body, an allergy, or an injury—things that can be demonstrated, realities that pay off because they lead us toward rational treatments. In psychiatry, rational treatments don't exist.

Before the age of biological psychiatry, those of us who are psychoanalysts were wildly enthusiastic about a parallel set of mythological pathologies, so enthusiastic that we thought we would eventually eliminate the social and psychological ills of all humankind. Incredibly, during the Cuban missile crisis, a group of American psychoanalysts, most of them senior members of departments of psychiatry at prominent universities, sponsored a movement to persuade John F. Kennedy, then the president, to be in psychoanalysis. He would then, you see, have been immune to folly.

Are you reminded of religion? Or of philosophy, which often claims to have pulled the rabbit out of the hat, to have discovered the foundation, the truth, the answer?

Freud and his psychoanalytic colleagues focused first on problems that had long been thought to be medical. The favourite target of the psychoanalysts was a problem that seemed to be a good example of something medical: conversion hysteria, a state in which patients have a cornucopia of paralyses, pains, vision problems, and swallowing disorders (no medical pathology has ever been found). Gradually, as psychoanalysts expanded their work, they took on the anxious, those who fret and organize (obsessives and compulsives), and depressives.

Eventually they took on the fully mad. It began to seem clear that, in the best of all possible worlds, *everyone*—including criminals and children, and especially psychiatrists and presidents—ought to be psychoanalyzed.

With the turn to biology, we again hoped we were going after examples of medical pathology. The favourites were schizophrenia, serious depression, and mania. Keen on emulating our psychoanalytic predecessors, as we gelled our convictions, we expanded our work to include the anxious, the intensely fretful, the super-organized, and the depressed. Like our psychoanalytic ancestors, we'd stumbled upon the bounty of speculative fancy, and began to take aim at criminals, smokers, gamblers, cross-cultural matters, and so on ad infinitum. Perhaps, instead of everyone being in analysis, all of us should take twenty milligrams of Prozac daily? Wild statements about invisible biological abnormalities do have a payoff, of course; they give birth to what Nietzsche called *conceptual mummies.* But to gauge improvement, cure, or change, something must exist that can be changed, and unfortunately for my credulous colleagues, conceptual mummies are figments of our imagination and are therefore not candidates for change. The patient's opinion doesn't count; anecdotes or testimony about "doing better" and "being cured" were as rampant five hundred years ago as they are today, and also, I assume, when cavemen walked the earth.

Despite the absence of pathology or evidence of change, when psychiatrists give drugs, electroshock treatments, and psychotherapies, patients and their families bestow accolades on us that we'd be fools to take at face value. Patients who believe they have been cured of something will be uneasy about what I've just said, as will colleagues whose careers depend on convincing the world that real psychiatric diseases exist. The madness-is-a-disease idea has become professionalized, a status that makes the belief in psychiatric diseases sacred, something divinized, and when science challenges a sanctified idea, it's heresy. My shrewdest critics will pose the most difficult question I'm up against: "Why rail against a benign fraud, a fertile falsehood, a community-building belief?" More harshly put, the question is whether something that makes people feel better should trump truth, even if it offers temporary comfort. With absolute conviction, here is my stand, a stand in favour of double-think and ambiguity:

1. I'm determined that psychiatrists should stand foursquare against pretense. That's because the psychiatric business is about honesty and frank talk about things people usually avoid, including bad breath, money, sex, and cowardice.

2. I'm determined to go along with any pretense, willing to use every trick in the book to help our patients, disdain truth at all costs, happy to help by giving a blessing, making a gesture, performing a ritual or magic—as long as these things don't remove civil rights or have nasty drug side effects and it is not implied that patients have biological or psychological abnormalities (point two is not natural to me, but helping people isn't sacred).

THE BEST SPECULATION we can come up with is to say that a psychiatric patient's way of life is one in which he himself still has a hand, a speculation that allows for hope; when things go sour, the mad, the unhappy, and the peculiar—any one of us, in fact—might have a change of heart about the directions we've chosen. *It's the only hope we've got.* This has nothing to do with the stupid idea that madness and suffering are free choices. Someone who lives in an extremely odd way does so for enormously complicated reasons, much more complicated than when it's said that people are depressed, nervous, or insane because of (imaginary) abnormal chemicals, genes, or brains. Life is more of a muddle than such simplistic explanations suggest, and change is more complicated still. Whether our patients are following a rocky path, live strange lives, or are trapped in a waking nightmare, many, as they always have, will stick to their unhappy ways. With or without pills, psychotherapy, or electric shocks, our only hope is that something internal will shift, that some psychiatric patients will change the direction of their lives. In this process, psychiatrists have always played a part.

When *Daggers of the Mind*,[1] my book about the placebo effect, was published, the reaction was colourful: columnists denounced me, enthusiasts wanted to join me in bringing down psychiatry, a television date was cancelled, and there was a referral to www.moronsabound.com.

---

1 Gordon Warme, *Daggers of the Mind: Psychiatry and the Myth of Mental Disease* (Toronto: House of Anansi Press Inc., 2006).

(A few days later the moronsabound fellow sent an apology. Had he changed his mind after reading more of my book? His website is now gone.) Extravagant reactions when doubts are raised make one suspicious, especially the strong reactions I get when I say that no objective evidence of psychiatric disease has ever been demonstrated. I do my best to respond archly: "Why not give me the evidence?" This retort is for the colleague who claims that her theories are scientific. Before she answers, I suggest she think carefully about the following questions:

Is there a way your theory can be proved wrong—refuted, in other words? For example, if you say depression is caused by chemical *X* in the brain, and chemical *X* isn't found, then the theory is refuted, right? You biology guys often say this, that depression is caused by abnormal brain chemicals, but where is the chemical? Which chemical do you have in mind? Cancer patients have cancer cells in their bodies every time; diabetic patients metabolize sugar abnormally every time; influenza patients have the influenza virus in their body every time; patients with glaucoma have high pressure inside the eyeball every time. As a scientist, you know that your theory must be evidence-based and falsifiable. If it isn't, the only thing you've got is metaphysics, religion, or superstition—all three being pretty well the same thing. Although I'm a clinician and not a scientist, even I know that. Don't you see that your thinking is identical to that of mediaeval priests, those who explained odd behaviour by saying it was caused by a demon whose existence they couldn't prove? That the only difference is the name: they called the demon Mephistopheles, Satan, or Splendiletto; you call yours Abnormal Chemical. I'm not teasing you. Your thinking is, really and truly, identical to that of ancient and modern demonologists; you *are* a demonologist.

The biological psychiatrists are determined that their use of the scientific method (*in theory*, that's what they use; in fact, they don't follow even rudimentary scientific rules) validates their diagnoses and their treatments, except that the desired validation has never happened. Therefore, what biological psychiatrists tell us about mental disease counts for nothing. What psychologically oriented psychiatrists tell us about mental disease counts for something, but not very much, since the latter rely on soft humanistic methods (biography, analogy, soft evidence) that support but cannot prove their diagnoses and their treatments to be right or wrong. Since these two kinds of psychiatrists represent mutually cancelling points of view, these two interpretive communities—these tribes, these cults—must debate the matter. We might hope that such a debate would settle things, but what gets "proved" is usually a matter of who is the better rhetorician.

Because they convince people they can cure things, the biologists of today often win the public relations debate. Seventy years ago, psychological psychiatrists also promised cures, and in those days, were winners in the public relations debate. Because they no longer exploit the word *science*, using soft persuasion instead, psychological psychiatrists now lose the debate. Because the biologists' territory is proof, and since they have none, nowadays they definitely lose the evidence debate; because the psychologists' territory is poetic and humanistic, they win the heart-and-souls debate, but only with the humanist and literary crowd. Many insecure humanist psychiatrists assuage their hurt feelings by scorning science; yet others do the opposite, make the preposterous claim that they *also* use the scientific method. Science and poetry be damned, all too often the outcome of such debates depends on political persuasion, just as the outcome of debates between religious fundamentalists and scientists depends on political persuasion—the true nature of science and poetry be damned.

Everyone knows that we humans kid ourselves. The great mendacities are not those of officials, fools, and charlatans; rather, they are the ones committed by you and me. I know for sure that I lie—especially to myself. Having experimented with various masks, all of us, including psychiatrists, settle on a mask or identity, believe in it, and expect others to believe it too. Because every psychiatrist deceives herself in one way or another, paying attention to her own self-blinding behaviour is central to her work, so central that, lest she hoodwink herself, she must think about her every reaction to her patients, her every comment, diagnostic thought, and recommendation. Because self-deception never ends, she is like everyone else—she never gets things exactly right.

It is said that an arrow of fire transfigured Saint Teresa of Ávila. Her statue, Bernini's *The Ecstasy of Saint Teresa*, stands in the Santa Maria della Vittoria chapel in Rome. Instead of being transfigured by modern medicine and good sense, hers is a story of ecstasy. The statue commemorates a dream described by Saint Teresa in her autobiography. Beside her in the chapel, holding a golden arrow, is an angel. She describes her experience of religious ecstasy in her encounter with the angel as follows:

> I saw in his hand a long spear of gold, and at the iron's point there seemed to be a little fire. He appeared to me to be thrusting it at times into my heart, and to pierce my very entrails; when he drew it out, he seemed to draw them out also, and to leave me all on fire with a great love of God. The pain was so great, that it made me moan; and yet so surpassing was the sweetness of this excessive pain, that I could not wish to be rid of it. The soul is satisfied now with nothing less than God. The pain is not bodily, but spiritual; though the body has its share in it. It is a caressing of love so sweet which now takes place between the soul and God, that I pray God of His goodness to make him experience it who may think that I am lying.[2]

No need to be shy about it—she is lying to herself and to us. Unless we want to join in on this mendacity, it's obvious what's going on: Saint Teresa is having an orgasm (Lacan's first reaction upon seeing the statue was, "She's coming"). The ecstatic look on the face of her statue mirrors that of Kripalu Maharaj, the guru whose orgasm I described in chapter 17. So maybe this is another treatment style—poetic, useless, thrilling.

St. Teresa radiates ecstasy, drama, and sex—her preferred version of change or transformation, analogous to but different from what many modern psychiatrists hope for. It may be about the need for an overwhelming experience, an arrow of fire. We all know this and have experienced it: mad love, an inspiring teacher, a Diego Rivera mural that wakens us to the horrors of the Spanish conquest of Mexico—experiences that, when they happen, move us, mark us. Certain diseases are like that—they progress to a crisis followed by one of two outcomes: resolution of the illness or, alternatively, a downhill course and death. If you read a bodice-ripper, you'll realize that love is also like that: it progresses to a crisis, followed by one of two outcomes: resolution through marriage or, alternatively, suffering and spiritual death.

---

2 *The Autobiography of St. Teresa of Ávila: The Life of St. Teresa of Jesus.* No publisher listed, but available at Indigo.ca, at Amazon.ca, and in any reference library, translated by David Rehak in 2013.

ONCE UPON A time, mythology and religion were our sublime truths, at another, realism, at yet another, romanticism. Nowadays it's liable to be modernism. To this list I could add democracy, liberty, and political correctness. If arranged in certain ways, such lists can be mistaken for a progression, a series of advances, but they are not. Nor do our patients "advance." We say they get better—patients often agree—but it's not true; although they may be different, only a moralist would say they are better. Nor does art progress or advance: I got teary-eyed when I saw the seventeen-thousand-year-old wall paintings in the Lascaux Caves, just as I'll get teary-eyed over this year's version of the *Romeo and Juliet* ballet. But I won't be teary-eyed over the ballet because of some weird notion that "art has advanced." Although they may change, music, dog farts,[3] and sex don't advance either.

Variations in art are in fashion in one era, forgotten for a while, and in accord with human whim, reborn in another era, just as psychiatric tastes come and go. For years, paintings of "reality"—people, still lifes, scenes—were thought to be supremely beautiful, and despite my worry that this proves I am an old fuddy-duddy, I admit that I don't like the modern tendency to abstraction. If I say that abstraction has gone too far, that art has been corrupted by drips and smears and used toothpaste tubes glued to a canvas, I may be wrong and I may be right—except art has no objective standard by which it can be judged. The paintings I find thrilling are old-fashioned: portraits, a broken fence, a merry-go-round, the aftermath of a massacre. The visual art I like is always a mimesis, a reproduction of something real rather than an abstraction, especially if it's a person. Yet the geometric ornamentation of the Blue Mosque in Istanbul and the Alhambra in Granada thrill me too, as do lush Orthodox churches and Gothic cathedrals.

---

3 Some will think I ought to apologize for using a vulgar fart analogy, but if I apologize and explain it away you'll sleepily carry on with your reading. And with a patient, if I apologize and rationalize something, he can also sleepily carry on. But if I *don't* apologize, he may be annoyed, the situation slightly disrupted. And if he's annoyed, he can notice something, the *circumstances* under which he gets annoyed. That's usual, but if, when I neither apologize nor explain, he admires me, it would be a counterintuitive response that would certainly catch my attention—and *his* attention if I can get him to notice what he's doing. It's one of my rules of psychiatry: "never apologize, never explain."

If I say that Schönberg's music is horrible, that he made a misstep with his twelve-tone row, no one can show me to be wrong; there is no standard, only varying subjective tastes. Lots of art is weird (weird according to what standard?) and always has been: African masks, sculptures of Mayan gods, clay figures of women with grossly exaggerated vulvas and breasts, or men with enormous penises. So when some of us say that traditional European art was beautiful and modern abstract art is ridiculous, we're wrong. As long as a group agrees that it's art, it's art—just as, if a group says something is a psychiatric treatment, voila, it's a psychiatric treatment.

As you can see, both art and people puzzle me, just as they puzzle you. So what's this got to do with psychiatry? The easy answer is that the artist, the madman, and the criminal are first cousins, all three being unconventionalists. But it's more complicated than that, so let me come at it in a roundabout way.

Parents raise children to do the right thing, to be conventional, to eat with a fork and knife, to wash, to say please and thank you. But when I became a grandfather, I found that I didn't act like a parent; instead, I corrupted my grandchildren, just a little bit. At my cottage on holidays, my grandchildren and I had secrets. In the spirit of naughtiness, while their parents were sleeping late in the morning, I gave them tiny cups of coffee, strictly against the rules. And when Miles was told he couldn't have another bedtime story and cried broken-heartedly, I didn't entirely take the side of the disciplining parent. Later that night, I snuck into his room and told him a story. I didn't *read* a story—even I have scruples—I only *told* a story. Mothers are usually conventional, sticking to doing what's the right thing, but fathers, just a bit, act like subversive grandparents and subversive uncles and aunts—they fart for their children.

This is the dichotomy I set up in chapter 16—the distinction between problems and mysteries. Although men are typically thought of as impulsive problem solvers, in the context of family and children it is more accurate to say this: parents, especially mothers, stand for problem solving, good sense, and practicality, whereas grandparents, uncles, and aunts—and to some extent fathers—stand for complexity, ambiguity, and variety. Parents bring up children to be sensible and to fit in, whereas grandparents teach that rules aren't absolute, that iron discipline is not only silly, but life defeating. Preachers on television teach the sensible line; comedians teach the unconventional line. Most of the time, yes, follow the rules and act conservatively; at other times, experiment and take risks.

The further analogy, the one I'm trying to get you to think about, is with art—including psychiatry (psychiatry is neither art nor science; it is a specialized social practice, a medical practice, but *art* is a good metaphor for psychiatry, especially for psychiatrists like me who are half-artist wannabes). Most of the time, traditional, conventional art predominates: novels that tell clear stories (stories we vaguely know already because we've read dozens of such novels), portraits, seascapes, and still lifes. But some of the time, art does otherwise—it's experimental, tries out abstraction, strange sounds, sculptures made out of garbage, novels like Virginia Woolf's *The Waves* or James Joyce's *Ulysses* that jump all over the place looking at the detritus of life.

When someone is in trouble, the same idea comes into play. Friends and family do the traditional thing—they behave sympathetically ("Oh, you poor thing," "He actually said that? Tell him to go to hell," or "Let's have a drink."). But sometimes tradition doesn't work (traditional paintings get boring; you've listened to Beethoven's *Fifth Symphony* too often; cornflakes and milk for breakfast have become passé), so something else is called for. And that's where the psychiatrist comes into the story. Although in emergencies she acts to cool things off in a very conventional way—reassurance, advice, some pills, a polite kick in the arse—in the back of her mind she knows that many patients have had enough of platitudes, advice, and bromides: with those patients she aims to eventually turn things upside down, subvert her patient's way of life, reinvent what's going on in unexpected ways. When she does this, the psychiatrist is a modern, therefore revolutionary artist who wants to paint Guernica, riff on "My Funny Valentine" in a way never done before. She's not Picasso, nor is she Miles Davis, but as a hard-working doctor she does her best. Some would say this is progress. I say that it is a modern but currently a fading taste in psychiatry.

Although interested in novel ideas, my favourite psychiatrist is wary of gimmicks: flashing neon lights, colon irrigation, and deep-brain stimulation aren't in her repertoire. These things "work," of course, but they might not suit people who think of themselves as sophisticated, and since they want to be accepted by both fancy and ordinary people—derelicts and booze artists too—psychiatrists tend to choose "scientific" things like drugs. Despite my prejudgments, many working-class people, panhandlers, and crooks share my interest in myths, Nietzsche, and novels about the detritus of life. If I tell my street-lady patient the story of Jacob stealing the blessing from Esau, she is interested, and she understands that giving the blessing to the second son is a moral dilemma worth thinking about, analogous to her awareness that being the favourite child can be problematic. In contrast, I find lots of things hokey that socially privileged people can be interested in: diets, exercise, yoga, meditation, and so on. The point is that, like art, *psychiatry does not progress, nor is one treatment better than another.*

Therefore, a manifesto: Leonardo da Vinci painted with as much talent as Picasso, Romeo was as fine a lover as James Bond, and Socrates argued as skilfully as Noam Chomsky. Like art, the act of love, and talented quarrelling, *psychiatry does not progress.*

This point bears repeating: as opposed to science, art does not advance and improve, and psychiatry, a social practice to which I'm now applying the metaphor of art, also does not advance and improve. *King Lear* is great literature, but *The Iliad*, written millennia earlier, is just as great, as is *Death of a Salesman*, written 450 years later. Rather than being a scientific discovery, Socrates's idea that the unexamined life is not worth living is an artistic statement made by a genius. Since it is not a hard fact, it has only one purpose: it makes us think. Freud was also a genius who made artistic statements; like Socrates, his statements aren't the "truth" but they make us think. Science and mathematics, on the other hand, grow and evolve, but since psychiatric practices are not scientific or mathematical, the treatments recorded almost four hundred years ago in Burton's *Anatomy of Melancholy* were as effective then as today's treatments are now. But since they are not in fashion, the treatments Burton described wouldn't work today.

Be it postmodern, modern, impressionist, or traditional, most art is ordinary. Only a fraction of it stands up over time. The same goes for psychiatry—most of its methods are not and have not been good art, as evidenced by the fact that most of the stuff we try out eventually ends up in the garbage can. But what if I'm wrong? What if lots of bad art has endured in the public imagination through inertia, fashion, or snobbery? Since there is no objective test for what is good art, there's no way of telling. As for psychiatry: light therapy, highfalutin talk, and antipsychotics have lasted and *will* last, their effectiveness equal to that of Lydia Pinkham's Pink Pills for Pale Ladies. That is to say, many patients will have an opinion that the pills help, just as in 1933 a majority of Germans were of the opinion that Hitler would make the best chancellor. Opinion is worth little, and it certainly isn't scientific—although, to my horror and amazement, psychiatric researchers think it is.

Saying that crazy and depressed people have abnormal brains has also been credulously accepted for thousands of years, and even though some patients are content to accept that idea and the treatments based on it, this particular myth of the abnormal brain must be strongly opposed. Why? Because that belief, that particular *fashionable* belief, leads to dangerous treatments like trepanning of the skull, lobotomies that tear out chunks of the brain—the "originator" of lobotomy won the Nobel prize in 1949—and the prescribing of dangerous drugs whose benefits are limited. Treatments are the same old magical themes of healing: taking something in the mouth, talking, scarifying (cutting, burning, shocking) the body, purging oneself, submitting to a shaman's opinion, pulling oneself together, taking a sea voyage.

The psychiatrist worth her salt does her best to give up on that stuff, not because it doesn't help, but because those who visit her have already tried all those things or have been advised to try all those things. She does her best to be artistic, to create collages out of what her patient does and doesn't tell her. I wish that three things were forbidden: first, doing harm (many drugs); second, telling the patient he is being "treated" (except as a tactical measure to get him through a rough spot); and third, defining him as a less than complete citizen (a person who should lose his civil rights, someone with a diseased brain).

If my patient is boring and pedantic, I torment him with drama and hyper-reality, including bafflement at his diligent avoidance of delight and fireworks; if he's dramatic and histrionic, I'm the one who becomes diligent, feeds him rational metaphors including reminders that he'll hate such metaphors and raising the question of why he avoids the rationally interesting. (I confess that my own weakness is to intervene rationally even when I ought to be a bit histrionic. I shouldn't be bland when pointing things out; I should try to exaggerate more, to spring things on my patient as a surprise, verbal tricks that make the idea more real than the original observation.) In other words, instead of thinking her patient must progress and develop, the psychiatrist is interested in the immediate, the present, and she therefore relies on two styles of intervention:

1. Duplication, pastiche, parody, satire, spoof, tender mockery, amusement, and horrified recognition (in homage to Louis C.K., Judy Holliday, and Jacques Lacan, I wish I could do this better).
2. Cold logic (Freud emphasized logic, but because he had a wonderfully imaginative mind, let slip many wild ideas).

The psychiatrist's idea is that getting better really means getting wise to the tricks that, by manipulating words and symbols and memories, we all play on ourselves.

I trust in the value of Albrecht Dürer's art for three reasons: my naïve pleasure in it, the judgments of experts, and because it has held the loyalty of many people over a long period of time—its historical staying power, the consensus of the ages. None of these reasons are decisive and none mean that Dürer's art is fundamentally or essentially good; they just mean that it's to the taste of people like me and the fanatics/ideologues/tribalists I want to team up with. The historical staying power of Dürer's art means only that it's a Western tradition. I strongly believe it is good art, but I shouldn't be dogmatic because it's just another of the signifiers that can be latched onto—and clung to—in my culture. Taste in art is only a taste—more slightingly, a fashion—and neither universal, permanent, nor absolute.

I approve of the "cure" by talking or insight for the same reasons: my naïve pleasure in participating in that cure, the intellectual arguments I can mount on its behalf, and its historical durability. I also approve of the talking cure because many unhappy people want it, hoping to talk with a culturally recognized expert. The opinion of Socrates and his successors, up to and including Freud, that the unexamined life isn't worth living, can therefore be endorsed—carefully—carefully because proponents of cures abound, and every believer thinks her version of cure to be sublime. But not me. I find it sublime to *not* believe in the sublime, find it wise to not know things for sure. If a fool practises the talking cure without reservation or some degree of skepticism, she can do harm; pills and potions are powerfully traditional but can have dreadful metabolic effects. The placebo effect makes us think it's legitimate to intrude on the body, to do things that are awful or ridiculous like bloodletting, cold packs, wet packs, and so on. In these cases, the family and the doctors often think the patient is better, and surprisingly the patient often agrees. Unless, of course, the insane person isn't treated at all, instead given special status. At Delphi, for example, madwomen were appointed to be seers—the Pythia—able to foresee the future; Charles Manson, interviewed on YouTube, is obviously insane, but was appointed by his followers to be their prophet.

Instead of writing about the thinking of the mad, James Joyce wrote in a mad language, "Finnegans-Wake-ese": a red rose becomes a red nose; a phoenix becomes a finish; a funeral becomes a fun-for-all. "Hail Mary, full of grease, the lard is with thee," he tells us, and "Wipe your glosses with what you know," all puns based on unexpected analogies. To complaints that his puns were trivial, Joyce answered with another pun: "Yes, some of my puns are trivial, and some are quadrivial." He was referring to the subjects studied in mediaeval universities: the Trivium—rhetoric, grammar, and logic—and the Quadrivium—arithmetic, geometry, astronomy, and music. It's precisely what a madman might say, except that the insane man speaks this way to persuade us to view him as bizarre and alien. Joyce, on the other hand, had a literary purpose, to persuade us of something important: intolerance of odd usage must be reconsidered. The sentence bears repeating:

Intolerance of odd usage must be reconsidered.

The preferred explanation of how Joyce came up with Finnegans-Wake-ese is that he dipped into his depths, his unconscious, into the seething cauldron kept at bay during ordinary, sane life. This is a metaphor, of course, but not an apt one because art is not primitive. When Joyce writes in unfamiliar language, he's not tapping into some unknown, mysterious, primitive mind, an imaginary cavern populated by warded-off ideas, freaks, and dwarfs. To suggest this is to ape mediaeval cartographers whose maps, at the boundaries of the known world, portrayed monsters and demons. Like the madman, the artist creates new forms. The barmy and the bard use novel language, the madman for one purpose, the artist for another. Neither Joyce nor the madman have sunk into infantilism or animalism or into the primitive. The only thing they've done is taken on artistic ways that some will call primitive and others will call advanced, even though they're neither.

A good work of art makes us think. When I see a painting by Rembrandt or Vermeer, I'm curious. "How the devil did he pull this off, those eyes, the stain on that wall, that pearl?" Or if I see a Picasso cubist painting, "Why did he do it that way? What the devil is it all about?" And as I listen to the ending of a Wagner opera, I'm baffled. "How does a human being create musical endings that stir me up like this, leave me reeling?" The answer is that the artist, whether she created her work three thousand years ago or three days ago, *makes us think*, which is exactly what the psychiatrist ought to do; her unexpected comments aim to get her patient thinking. Museums in Europe are filled with religious paintings: crucifixions, annunciations, nativity scenes. These paintings have little effect on me, but five hundred years ago they would have stirred people to do what art is supposed to do: make them think about God and life and how they live. Art that doesn't stir us up is like a psychiatrist who says, "Take this pill."

We extrude the mad from polite society, not because they are primitive, but because their odd language and unconventional opinions unnerve us. Psychiatrists ought to respond to the mad by thinking hard about what they tell us; all too often we respond by trying *not* to think at all about what they tell us, in one way or another, shutting them up. We humans are a demanding species; we require of one another that we conform, obey rules that, although not codified, are strict. Most of us discourage unusual thinking when we run into it, often by way of strong body-language responses. At our worst, we psychiatrists ward off discomfiting thinking coercively, all too often with drugs, euphemized as therapeutic bullets. We're even ambivalent about ordinary—as opposed to crazy—creativity: some find unexpected creativity alarming and in need of censorship; others celebrate creativity as refreshing, hopeful, and to be encouraged. I suspect that the creative strangeness of the insane has been designed by them to provoke the former reaction—alarm. And it's all done using archetypes understood by all able-minded members of our culture.

20

Unweaving the Rainbow

One unerring mark of the love of truth is not entertaining any proposition with greater assurance than the proofs it is built upon will warrant.

JOHN LOCKE

THE RAINBOW IS the beautiful daydream of psychiatry, the theories of marvellous chemicals and complexes so many of my colleagues swoon over, the metaphors they mistake for facts. Although such theories have no payoff, like rainbows, they enthrall us, and many of my fellow priests, shamans, and psychiatrists use their prestige to convince the world that these imaginary entities actually exist. Were we to follow the scientific method, we couldn't make this mistake, but many of my colleagues won't let go, hanging on to hypotheses even though they fulfill no scientific criteria. Defective neurotransmitter activity in the brain could, if it existed, be discovered, but bad object relations (psychiatric jargon for bad human relationships) can never be discovered because the phrase is nothing more than a moral judgment. Presupposing damage and abnormality when someone acts in an unconventional way is analogous to sexism and prejudice. If you tell me my brain is abnormal, it's an insult: "Are you brain-dead or something?" or "Have you got a screw loose?" or "Are you soft between the ears?"

There are two legitimate approaches to understanding. The first is scientific explanation—discovering causes, in other words—which is enlightening and unequivocal. The second is mental and social talk, interpretation, and the redescription of what's going on, including showing connections and patterns, an approach that is typically metaphoric and imaginative, one used by psychiatrists, novelists, anthropologists, poets, and artists. Mental and social talk is also illuminated by collecting evidence, by noticing historical patterns, and by quoting authorities whose opinions are both respected (many fools are respected) and whose work has survived careful scrutiny (careful scrutiny isn't common). Both scientific explanation by way of causes and understanding people through interpretation, analogies, and links are important medical methods for understanding patients, but the first, science, works only with patients who have biological abnormalities. Under the Nazi regime, the German public believed their "experts" too, the so-called scientists who measured skulls and noses with callipers and tape measures, and who "proved" that Jews, homosexuals, and gypsies were biologically different from the rest of us. It's tempting to dismiss the German scientists of the 1930s and '40s as old-fashioned fools, but at that time, German science, especially medical science, was the gold standard.

Another preposterous example comes from the time of apartheid in South Africa. Millions of citizens were assigned to a "race," either white, black, coloured (racially mixed), or Asian (Indian). If it was not immediately obvious to which race a person should be assigned, the distinction between black and coloured might be decided by the pencil test. The person was asked to put a pencil behind his ear; if the pencil stayed in place, he was assigned to the category of black, with dire consequences for his future life. This piece of idiocy depended on believing that the ears of blacks fit more tightly to the head than do the ears of people from other races. And currently we hear about the current gold standard of Western psychiatry, now spreading all over the world: there are "soon-to-be-discovered" abnormalities.

The rules of science can prevent such errors, rules that are not complicated. Scientific explanation, the rules say, tells us the cause of something so consistently that its existence can be predicted with confidence. But prediction doesn't mean a scientific theory is perfect or final; it means only that for now the theory is a good one. As made clear by Karl Popper, the essential rule is that a scientific theory must be *falsifiable*; that is to say, the theory must be constructed in such a way that one can imagine a circumstance in which the theory can be proved wrong.[1] It's how science progresses: as time goes on, scientific theories become increasingly less reliable, and demonstrating the unreliability of established theories is a large part of the everyday work of the scientist. When they test theories, scientists are, among other things, trying to ferret out problems in their theories, setting the stage for scientific progress by replacing weaker theories with stronger theories. For example, the Copernican theory of the solar system replaces the Ptolemaic system; the theory of chemicals replaces the theory of humours; the theories of relativity replace Newtonian physics. As examples, let me use the abnormal-chemical-in-the-brain theory of depression and the Newtonian theory of the relationship between space and time:

- An abnormal chemical in the brain explains depression; Newtonian physics explains the relationship between space and time.
- No abnormal chemicals are found in the brain of a depressed person; the Michelson–Morley experiment demonstrates that the Newtonian explanation of the relationship between space and time is not correct.
- The biological theory of depression is refuted; the Newtonian theory of the relationship between space and time is refuted.
- No better (explanatory) theory of depression exists to take the place of the abnormal chemical theory; a better theory of the relationship between space and time, the special theory of relativity, exists and therefore replaces the Newtonian theory.

A scientist who doesn't follow these rules is a classicist without Greek, a parson without divinity, an English professor without Shakespeare, a psychiatrist who doesn't listen. For example, once it was realized that many cases of multiple sclerosis turned out to have no

1 Karl R. Popper, *Unended Quest: An Intellectual Autobiography* (Illinois: Open Court Publishing, 1976).

venous blockage in the neck, no doctor or scientist would believe that venous blockage causes multiple sclerosis.

Freud indulged in wishful thinking, believed that his psychoanalytic method truly gave him access to objective data. His intellectual charisma earned him many disciples, and his way of practising eventually became widespread. Because she has no more data than Freud had, the modern psychiatrist also does something scientifically improper, so improper that it's more accurate to say she does something ridiculous: she announces that "very soon, we will discover objective data." This claim is a superstitious conviction, no different from saying, "Very soon, we will see the second coming of Christ" or "Very soon, we will arrive at the end of history" or "very soon, I will have bad luck if I walk under a ladder or spill salt without immediately throwing a pinch of it over my shoulder." In the meantime, while waiting for the miraculous appearance of evidence (Christ? the end of history? bad luck?), the psychiatrist does what has always been done—she talks to her patients. And she does neither physical examinations nor does she order diagnostic tests. This ought to mean there is nothing for the psychiatrist to do except to talk to her patients, but these days she commonly does try to do something more than that—she gives drugs. Without objective data, no one can build a scientific theory, but just the same, somehow unable to control herself, the mortal psychiatrist invents brain theories as inglorious and imaginary as Freud's bad theories (he had amazingly good ones too, but they were not scientific), empty theories she uses as a rationale for giving powerfully disabling drugs to her patients.

Were I to say pneumonia is a brain disease, you'd think me odd. Yet once in a while, when examined, people with pneumonia do have an abnormality—an *incidentaloma*—in their brain X-ray, an abnormal EEG, or other minor neurological findings. According to the logic I'm complaining about, this could be considered "suggestive evidence" that pneumonia is caused by brain abnormalities—a conclusion that would make every doctor laugh. When a researcher—I'll call her Dr. X—notices that one of the patients in her schizophrenia research study has something odd in his brain, she is eager to believe that this is evidence that schizophrenia might be caused by an abnormal brain. Very quickly, however, she will find that the other schizophrenic patients in her research group rarely or never have the suspected abnormality, and her project will prove negative. Despite failures, Dr. X and her research-minded colleagues keep the faith, continue to believe their brain theories.

But in her clinical role, things are different. When not wearing her research hat, and when faced with one of her own schizophrenic patients who at a routine visit unexpectedly turns out to have signs of a brain abnormality, Dr. X will, I assume, contradict her research practices. Although in her theoretical work she's eager to find a brain cause for schizophrenia, with her own patient, if a brain lesion shows up, she will withdraw the diagnosis of schizophrenia! Obviously, the new diagnosis will be the abnormality that has been found: scar in the parietal lobe, tumour in the basal ganglia, cyst in the prefrontal cortex, infection of the meninges—whatever! These are, of course, solid, standard criteria of disease in the brain—but not of schizophrenia. When practising as a front-line doctor, she thinks properly. We all differ biologically, so anyone can have "abnormalities" here or there, now and then. Besides, if my colleagues are really convinced that psychiatric disorders are physical diseases, they would do what doctors from all other specialties do: physical examinations.

Studies of my brain can isolate the source of many reflexes (automatic actions of the body over which I have no control), but there's nothing that will pin down what language I speak, my behaviour, my sexual orientation, my marital status, or my interests. Nor can structures be located that will tell you whether I have or do any of the things that get called psychiatric disease. But there's no need to fret. Because you have been designed by evolution and by your rearing to be socially clever, able to intuit my purposes, interests, and intentions quickly and brilliantly, all you have to do is ask me about my sexual orientation, my marital status, and my interests, and you'll know. It's as simple as that. The same goes for craziness. Don't bother to examine my body; just have a conversation with me and you'll know right away whether I'm crazy. Anyone who thinks she can figure out these things by studying my brain is ridiculous; two hundred thousand years of evolution has designed humans to be somewhat more efficient than brain scans—a billion times more efficient. That's why talking is and always will be the primary instrument of the psychiatrist. You don't have to think about my brain for a nanosecond.

This, of course, is psychology, and in a strict sense psychology is not scientific. I'm lecturing in China in a few months, and I've arranged for my host to meet me at the airport. Using psychology, I strongly assume she will be there. Because psychology is presumptive rather than scientific, there is no guarantee. Some people might suggest that my *attitude* is scientific: I've had many experiences of arranging to meet someone, and usually the person who agreed to meet me has shown up—in other words, I have evidence. But only "usually." I don't approve of using the word *science* in this way because people assume that means something has been proved, and social actions, although guessable or probable, are not reliably predictable as are scientific predictions. You, I, and everyone else have had a lifetime of experience studying social behaviour, psychology, and we're all good at it.

IN ORDER TO make a causal, pseudo-scientific theory work, the psychiatrist must insist that her implausible theories are actually plausible. She must therefore invent absurd systems like *faculty theory*. Faculty theory postulates that the mind is made up of a bunch of mental structures called faculties: feeling, judging, thinking, impulse control, compliance, reliability. If a person says he caused the sun to rise this morning with his mind, his psychiatrist will say he has a defect in one of his mental faculties, his reality testing—although she doesn't say this if someone announces that God has blessed him, or that he has eaten the body and blood of Christ on Sunday morning. What she ought to say is simpler: the person who thinks he caused the sun to rise is saying something *unconventional*, while the person who speaks of being blessed and who claims to eat the body and blood of Christ is saying something *conventional*. When a talking psychiatrist says that someone has an ego weakness or a superego defect, or when a biologically oriented doctor says that someone has an abnormal chemical in his brain, she has joined in on a silly theory of missing parts.

Since no one has found any biological markers of psychiatric disorders, psychiatrists try hard to identify psychological markers. They have the idea that faculties have gone missing—for example, judgment, cognitive, or social "deficits." What they mean is that their patient can't do certain things like judging, thinking, and interacting socially. But if we study behaviour, we can come to no such conclusion, best demonstrated through an example. If I play Beethoven's *Moonlight Sonata* for you on the piano, it's obvious that my piano-playing faculty is intact. On the other hand, if I *don't* play the *Moonlight Sonata*, it doesn't mean my piano-playing faculty is damaged or absent. It means one of three things: I don't want to play the piano, I can't play it, or I want to deceive you about my ability to play the piano. I know I can write a book because I've done it several times, but if I don't write a book, I may well have the ability, despite the nonexistence of any book-writing activities. I don't go to brothels. This doesn't mean I couldn't go to a brothel, that I have a deficit in my brothel-going faculty. It means only that I opt not to go.

If I ask a patient to tell me where Albert Einstein came from, and he answers, "It's relative," he's obviously intending to give a peculiar answer. There is no deficit, only an unexpected answer, one that, if I consider my question to be a test, I could call a failure: "His information faculty is impaired." When one patient was asked, "What do fourteen and fourteen make?" he answered, "Well, about twenty-eight to forty-two." When I told this example to a colleague with whom I was debating, she said, "Yeah, but that particular patient is saying that on purpose." Exactly. That's the point of my example, that it's impossible to judge a social practice as a deficit because such answers are incomprehensible without the idea of *intent*. That the patient answers at all—even that he speaks—makes it clear that only by attributing intent can we make any sense at all of what someone says. Every psychiatrist is familiar with such "incorrect" answers, yet clearly the patient knows the "correct" answer. His cognitive "deficit" turns out not to be a deficit after all. Faced with this strange logic, the psychiatrist is liable to say the patient *cannot* give the correct answer. When she says this, she is wrong: as distinct from *can*not, her patient *does* not give the correct answer. No defect, only difference.

Such answers may provoke or annoy the psychiatrist, but if she tells herself the patient is abnormal, has "deficits," she can spare herself the discomfort of being annoyed; instead, she can say she is "detecting pathology." I suspect that the decision to switch from social adjudication to diagnostic pathology also depends on thinking that it's not nice to say, "The way this patient answers questions pisses me off," "This answer is very funny," or "He's obstructionistic and shrewd." One of my reactions to such social practices is a tentative suspicion that the crazy person gives peculiar answers precisely so the psychiatrist and all the other people he runs into won't have ordinary reactions to him. The patient who makes peculiar judgments may well have the capacity to make conventional ones, but doesn't opt to do it when he talks to his doctor—or to anyone else. What the doctor ought to say is that her patient makes peculiar judgments, and does so for unknown reasons.

The same goes for cognition, judgment, and social style. To conclude that the person has a "deficit" in his judgment function is to make a medical analogy, a *weak* medical analogy, hoping that judgment can be compared to producing insulin, something that the pancreases of most people can do and the pancreases of diabetic people cannot. Because any human act can be (incorrectly) judged as reflecting a deficit, in the psychological realm this doesn't work. Were we to permit such an analogy, the driver who runs a red light could be said to have a deficit in his brake-pedal-depressing function, the humourist a deficit in his solemnness function, and the lover a chastity deficit. I'm inclined to say that the thinking of those professionals who argue that psychiatric patients have psychological deficits falls into the same category as the thinking of schizophrenic patients: disconcerting, bizarre, peculiar, and—yes—very funny. Or is it a deficit in their ability to follow scientific rules? Like any other form of madness, the naïveté of psychiatrists who think and argue this way is also not a disease.

A BIOLOGICAL CAUSAL theory of my behaviour is impossible. Because memories infuse, influence, and govern everything I do, the biological encoding of my every memory would have to be identified—wherever that encoding might be. To explain my way of thinking about psychiatry, the biology of every aspect of my participation in my culture would have to be nailed down, my lifelong nutritional experiences, how my tissues metabolized them and transformed them into body/brain tissue, plus the air I've breathed, the pills I've taken, my sexual experiences—and so on ad infinitum. And it wouldn't just be a study of my brain; my every experience is also embedded in every organ, muscle, limb, and skin surface of my body. Every erotic touch I've experienced—in the first year of my life alone I experienced a million erotic touches, and plenty more as an adult—has become part of the architecture of my skin and my brain and my soul, so there'd be a lot of tissue analysis to do.

An insane reductionist would say yes, that is the challenging task faced by psychiatry, and we've just got to plug away. Such an explanation would have to account for an infinity of factors for everything, for the most trivial nuance of behaviour, including why I used the word *nuance* in the previous clause of this sentence. I used the word *nuance* because it's a neat word, I like it, it seemed to fit the bill, and it clicked for me—a literary click, a polemical click, an opinion not understood by those who want scientific explanations for everything. A true eliminative materialist would have to be a nutcase! Keen on reductionism, she would have to reduce my behaviour to brain tissues, then to chemicals, then to molecules, then to atoms, and finally to elementary particles like quirks and quarks and neutrinos. In recent years, this nonsense has become a search for the seat of consciousness. Would anyone be so obtuse to say that the seat of consciousness is in an elementary particle like a boson or a fermion? And as we move up the scale from elementary particles to the universe, who would say that consciousness is located in atoms (carbon, helium, or hydrogen), molecules (proteins, water, collagen), or body tissues (muscle, bone, neurons, or the clusters of neurons called nuclei or ganglia)? But many say that the *brain* is conscious, even though it's obvious that "consciousness" is a quality of a person, not of the mass of tissues called the brain.

WE HUMANS AREN'T scientific in our dealings with one another, nor do I think that, most of the time, we even have a scientific attitude. It's just talk, yak-yak, rational, passionate, conventional, whatever. When I talk about myself, I don't amputate my will or agency—*agency* being the capacity, condition, or will of a person to act or exert power. I say, for example, that I am typing these words. But this isn't as obvious or universal a practice as it might seem; an ancient Greek would have removed agency from *me* (that's what the "chemical" psychiatrists are doing) and said that my finger joints were typing these words. And were

I writing passionately and furiously, that same ancient Greek would have said that the gods had taken possession of me, that they, the gods, were typing these words. An idealist philosopher would beg to differ, saying that the idea that I am typing is nothing more than a perception or a conception in my mind or yours, while a materialist philosopher, also differing, would spell out the muscles, nerves, and brain correlates of my typing. These various opinions are known as *theories of agency*.

But attributing agency to the patient rather than to his brain or his complexes can lead to trouble. Certain doctors, in *thrall* to the free-will version of agency, have failed to understand that free will is only a theory, helpful in certain circumstances and not helpful in others. Theories are tools, good for some things and not others: I don't use a hammer to stir my soup, nor do I use my garden rake to dig a hole in my flowerbed. (This is the same philosophical error—stupidity—as the debate between biological causation and social speculation, except that I've used slightly different language. It's the error of believing that these two theories are in the same logical universe and therefore in competition with one another.) Those who overuse the theory of free will risk defining our patients as imposters and be tempted to say, "There's nothing wrong with you. It's all in your head. You're a faker. Get out of this clinic." Fifty years ago, I actually saw doctors do this. Because these doctors weren't paying attention, they didn't notice that, for example, histrionic behaviour is a statement that something has gone awry, is an alert, a signal directed to a doctor whose job description is to talk through issues. Although such patients "do" their histrionic behaviour, this is not the same as "doing it on purpose."

Most theories of agency have no psychiatric payoff. Because there's no evidence and no dividend, my ideal psychiatrist is only mildly interested in biology, astrology, demon possession, and psychic energy. To confound things, even personal agency doesn't have a payoff that's immediately obvious. What it does accomplish is offer hope, suggesting that because the patient has a hand in how he lives, change is possible. And because the psychiatrist keeps describing what the patient is doing, she enlists him into her campaign of curiosity. She might (briefly) be interested in unexpected theories, invoking ideas like this: "I guess it's your destiny to have no permanent woman in your life" or "Fate has dealt you a bad hand." The psychiatrist who invokes destiny and fate is speaking metaphorically, of course. What she means is that, although out of fashion, these notions help us to accept the heartaches and nuisances of life. And although she has, in effect, told her patient that he can't do anything about his problem with women, she doesn't really believe this and will therefore keep pushing him to think about how, when, where, and why he sabotages his dealings with women. Despite her determination that personal agency is to have priority, and because our language is flexible, interesting, and comprehensive, she's willing to talk about events in other ways.

Whether or not she thinks of him as having a hand in his suffering (the ill-conceived debate between free will and determinism), a doctor's creed ought to be that anyone who knocks on her door is signalling that something has gone wrong and deserves help. Outside of psychiatry, doctors may well cure something; within psychiatry, the vague word *help* is the only one that fits. The contorted quest to find causal explanations is nothing new, as seen in the following examples from Greek history.

Like modern psychiatrists, ancient Greeks believed they knew exactly what caused human actions, causes that made sense to them; twenty-five hundred years later, these causes sound preposterous. To the Greeks, every important action was performed, not by the individual as a product of his or her own will, but by the gods. Should a person win in battle, marry, or get home safely, for example, the cause was assigned to the realm of the spirit and the poetic—in other words, to the gods. For these sacred beliefs, they had no evidence. (Lesser actions also had causes, but these were rational and physical rather than godly. Instead of saying, "I walked across the field," the Greeks said, "My joints carried me across the field.") Because only the gods could be the cause of important things, old Priam told Helen that to him she was not and could not be the cause of the Trojan War. If Helen provoked Paris to carry her off, she did so in a state of *átē* (divine infatuation), a form of mental incapacity. The word *responsibility* made no sense to the ancients.

In Greek tragedy, the characters lived out dramatic events innocently, unaware of hidden causal forces the audience knew about. The audience knew because a chorus gave voice to the decisive causes for why Oedipus, Clytemnestra, and Helen behaved as they did—again, it was the gods. Sometimes, in addition to the chorus, puppets of gods were suspended over the stage. As the puppets approached the actors to exercise their tutelary, inspiring, and malignant powers, the crowd cheered or booed, just as we cheer or boo when Batman, the Joker, or the Penguin approach the scene of action.

When I went to see Wagner's *Ring Cycle,* I was told that I ought to study up. "Why so?" I asked. The answer was that the actions and singing tell only the surface story; things aren't as clear as they appear on the stage. In truth, I was told, Wotan, Brünnhilde, Siegfried, et al. stumble through their lives, clueless about the chaotic forces that are in play, causes that impel them to act as they do. Those hidden causes—should I begin to suspect brain chemicals and brain structures or perhaps mental complexes?—are revealed by Wagner's music, which is informational. It informs us of Dionysian truths—chaos, arbitrariness, intoxication—as important as the straightforward Apollonian story sequences apparent on the stage. Less explicitly, the musical score of a movie serves a similar purpose.

The mad tell us they act as they do because of voices, X-rays, laser beams, and poisons. Three centuries ago, they also included demons and spirits in their list of hidden causes, and they were as willing as neurobiologists, ancient Greeks, and Freudians to believe without evidence.

Modern biological psychiatrists happily agree with the mad that they act as they do because of abnormal chemicals and brain abnormalities, a conclusion they come to because of their own credulity—they believe what the mad tell them about poisons, X-ray effects on their brains, and rotting nerves. Bereft of evidence, these doctors are persuaded by their fanciful theories, so certain that they regularly invoke legal measures to apprehend, confine, and treat people who they believe have these mental "diseases."

Mediaeval doctors and priests also agreed with the mad that hidden causes lay behind their behaviour: demon possession, copulation with incubuses and succubuses, and pacts with Mephistopheles. In other words, having taken their patients' and parishioners' words at face value, they believed what the mad told them about the malignant effects of sex and demons. And occasionally there were strategically placed anomalies—moles and suggestive marks between the legs that were, as you will surely have realized, bite marks rather than variants. They invoked the then-current legal measures that authorized them to apprehend, confine, and treat these people. We moderns roast certain patients with ECT, anticipated in this practice by mediaeval priests who also arranged for the mad to be roasted—to death.

Yes, even today, psychiatry lives under the spell of make-believe rainbows. In this chapter, I hope I've shown why that rainbow needs to be unwoven.

21

Psychiatry minus the Humbug

The snake which cannot cast its skin has to die.
As well the minds which are prevented from
changing their opinions; they cease to be mind.
NIETZSCHE

I'M GETTING LONG in the tooth, so I've laid down my cards, allowed you to see what's in my hand. I guess the aphorist is right: the Owl of Minerva takes wing only at dusk. I've picked six main targets:

- The psychiatric tendency to talk to and about psychiatric patients as though they are passive victims of biological or mental flaws even though no flaws have ever been discovered.
- The neglect of the obvious, that the only things we can observe and the only things our patients can tell us about are their social practices (often unconventional, sometimes disturbingly so).
- The overuse of powerful drugs, most of which are nothing more than chemical shackles—poisons.
- Offering psychotherapy to individual patients for dozens or hundreds of hours, thereby giving a tremendous amount of psychiatric time to a small handful of patients, shrinking an already limited resource.

- The futility of psychiatric research, which, despite millions of dollars spent, has never come up with discoveries. Because our patients show no abnormalities upon which research could be done, psychiatry cannot come up with discoveries.
- The failure of the profession to emphasize that people find their greatest solace in being beguiled by inspiring leaders, doctors, gurus, and priests, some of whom, unfortunately, are fools or scoundrels.

Having done this as exuberantly and as critically as I could, I've changed, but my vision is only somewhat different—new metaphors for old, so to speak. Nevertheless, it should be clear that my vision remains very different from that of many of my colleagues. I've said my piece, and if others join in on this truth-telling project, psychiatry's delusions won't be as safe.

> It is true there is not enough beauty in the world.
> It is also true that I am not competent to restore it.
> Neither is there candour, and here I may be of some use.[1]

Except for the most distressed and strange cases (they'll still have to be in an institution), I want psychiatric problems to be taken care of by family doctors, hairdressers, bartenders, and neighbours; their tradition of playing that role and their native ingenuity should suffice. I don't want them to think they need special training, that they must take technical courses in interpersonal psychotherapy, cognitive behaviour therapy, anger management, and psychoanalysis. I want them to be wise old types, experienced citizens who have good sense to pass on. I know that some will blunder. They will, for example, tell unhappy wives to "Just go home and cook dinner!" or "Quit being your husband's servant!"—advice that, although it may sometimes hit exactly the right note, may on other occasions be arbitrary and sexist. Some of these counsellors will be empathy and/or tough-love aficionados, tactics I don't like, but because these tactics will be neutralized by different

---

1 Louise Glück, *October* (Louisville, KY: Sarabande Books, 2004).

messages unhappy people will get from friends, fitness trainers, and newspaper articles, they're harmless in everyday life. (The same tactics are, however, unforgiveable if dispensed by psychiatrists who haven't thought things over.) Most of the time, day-to-day advice will be just fine. Often, it will steer families toward caring for their own, but this is an option that will alienate and frighten families who are faced with the awful burden of taking care of deeply eccentric members. It's a difficult world for all, a lot harder for some.

I have to remind myself that psychiatry—sort of—works, just as, for example, the church and the priesthood once worked. When sick, people went to church and prayed, and when overwhelmed, they talked with the priest. In those great churches and cathedrals they also found beauty and grandeur. As is typical of all tastes, the attractions of the church—the priestly and the artistic—are changing and weakening; the sacred functions that once made churches necessary are neglected in favour of activities that resemble what goes on in a social club. What churches have abandoned has bifurcated: for art and beauty, people visit new temples called museums and galleries; for health and talking, they visit doctors and the temples called hospitals, complete with soaring atriums and plaques identifying not kings and princes but donors.

Like priests and modern doctors, psychiatrists no longer offer a sacred style, the thing that patients want and need. Dramatic psychiatric treatments have been demoted to routines carried out by prescription, no longer administered by senior and important-looking clinicians. Occasionally, I interview one of my student resident's patients (the resident sits in and watches), but I worry about the impact my unusual interviewing style has on the patient. Even many months later, the patient will ask my resident, "Who was that guy who interviewed me, the guy who spent so much time talking about my tattoo?" I worry because I've stolen from the resident the doctor idealization that would best have landed on her. Because I'm prone to folly like all people, I also enjoy the idea that I'm seen as a dramatic hero who can pass on to the resident the dirty job of unravelling the patient's idealization of me.

The irrational demand that psychiatrists do research has created a climate of scientism, a belief that we can objectively study diseases that don't exist, and that the human mind can be studied as though it is a *thing* like an elbow, a liver, or an eyeball. It's a mess, and my stridency gives away my concern and my annoyance. I'm most appalled that psychiatrists cooperate in locking up people who act crazy and have broken the law, thereby defining them as fools too stupid to face the consequences of their own deeds. I'm even more appalled that psychiatrists participate in locking up people who are crazy but have *not* broken the law. I also worry about drugs that come in handy occasionally but that can also do serious harm, and about strange treatments—they don't suit my preference for restraint—like ECT, light therapy, and deep-brain stimulation. There's no denying that psychiatrists also bring to their work kindness and human concern, and probably that's the best thing we do. But human concern is undermined by bad theories, scores of them, theories that multiply like black flies in the spring and lead to desperate attempts to give a definitive treatment, even though a definitive treatment doesn't exist.

But if many patients are happy with the treatments they receive, isn't that good enough? My answer is no. Too much tolerance and too much liberalism means going along with things that are bad. Of course, my way—endlessly decoding symbols, forever examining the motives of my patients—also leads into limbo, into a mind-cramp, so in the end, an opinion is called for. It's my rape metaphor, its last gasp, unrecognizable because it has a new shape—a strong attack on bigotry and authoritarianism and subjugation with drugs, a dream I have for psychiatry that hasn't yet come true.

What if the psychiatrist were to reject all diagnostic terms, instead used ordinary words like *nervous*, *crazy*, *manic*, *withdrawn*, *weird*, *obnoxious*, *hysterical*, *obsessive*, and *depressed*? This would help her to avoid thinking of her patient as a victim of disease, a view that encourages passivity and helplessness. Instead, the emphasis would be on thinking of the patient as the agent of his own life, not because he is, really and truly, the agent of his own life—agency is a theory, not a fact—but because there's a payoff. If the helping person insists that her client has a hand in how he lives his life, she can raise the question of whether he might rethink things; if treated as a full citizen, not slotted into a category that defines him as impaired or challenged, the patient will be freed of a malignant prejudice, the hierarchical opinion that he is the helper's inferior—inferior to a psychiatrist who is only another citizen.

What if the psychiatrist-in-training were to study comic books, sleaze, anthropology, philosophy, psychology, literature, music, and film (as part of my official psychiatric training, I had as in-residence teachers Isaac Bashevis Singer and Margaret Mead), and what if she also had to study the placebo effect, including examining reports of magical cures by quacks, priests, and shamans?

What if the psychiatric trainee were assigned her first patient on the day she began her training and, closely supervised, immediately began meeting with that patient for an hour five times a week, similar to the talking work I've described myself doing in earlier chapters? Offering such an intensive form of treatment is not practical—too expensive—so the patients who receive it would be fortunate special cases, able to have this service only because it is necessary for the student's training. As the student years pass, the trainee would do less of this work, and after being qualified she would rarely take on intensive cases. But in the meantime, she will have learned from Nietzsche to listen meta-psychologically:

> I want to learn more and more to see as beautiful what is necessary in things; then I shall be one of those who make things beautiful. *Amor fati*: let that be my love henceforth! I do not want to wage war against what is ugly. I do not want to accuse; I do not even want to accuse those who accuse. *Looking away* shall be my only negation. And all in all and on the whole: some day I wish to be only a Yea-sayer.[2]

As a meta-commentator, the psychiatrist sees only the cleverness and ingenuity of her patients' words, even if the patient acts against his own interests, is an eternal naysayer, or doesn't write the great Canadian novel. If she stays meta, the psychiatrist will find everything fascinating, her philosophical stance so powerful that, without neglecting suffering, her attitude will override suffering. And as her patients

---

2 Friedrich Nietzsche, "Why I Am So Clever," in *Ecce Homo: How One Becomes What One Is*, Section 10 (Oxford, UK: Oxford University Press, reissue edition 2009).

notice her attitude, they will take it on. Nietzsche the yea-sayer is capable of accepting reality just as it is. Nietzsche also insists on the same trick when he writes about "eternal recurrence." Here's how it would work: should you have to repeatedly live your life over again—and again and again—and were you to stand back and watch, you'd have no wish to change a single thing that happened, as engrossed by your failures and stupidities as by your triumphs. I, for example, would no longer regret breaking up with Carol G. in high school after only two weeks of dating. She was pretty and smart and had a cute figure. Miraculously, she let me touch her breasts. But were I to grab onto Nietzschean and proper psychiatric thinking, I'd be a yea-sayer about everything I've ever done and about everything that has happened to me; I'd be content with having broken up with Carol G.; I wouldn't even have to Google her. Yes, *amor fati*.

Although her patients will do most of the talking, I imagine the psychiatrist of the future making a careful commentary on things other people say only behind her patient's back. As though a participant in the *corrida de toros*, she would aim for absolute honesty, zero in on what we humans are often hypocritical about, on horror and sex, on death and the maiden, on stupidity and evil. Because advice and support are common courtesies freely offered by friends and family—even by strangers—the psychiatrist wouldn't bother with those, would instead devote her time exclusively to serious topics.

And since she can't predict human behaviour better than any other citizen—not very well, in other words—the psychiatrist would no longer make prophecies about dangerousness. Statistics don't count; psychiatric patients do kill more people than the public at large, but not as many as drunk drivers, yet no one argues that we should commit a drinking driver against his will because he has a statistical advantage in the killing stakes. Nor, since no one could possibly know this, would my ideal psychiatrist comment on whether an offender knows the nature and quality of his actions. Because the courts and the police have adopted the fashion of sending those accused of horrible crimes to psychiatrists—a fashion that is at best naïve political correctness and at worst evading doing their duty—they will definitely be disappointed in this recommendation.

The psychiatrist is like everyone else. She identifies with a variety of like-minded people, those in whom she can recognize tribal affiliations—intellectual, racial, linguistic, historic, through blood or geography or class—affiliations she will, of course, have in common with her very crazy patients but that are obscured or made invisible by crazy talk and behaviour. Since the qualities in her mad patient the psychiatrist could identify with are masked by bizarreness and incomprehensibility, it's hard or impossible for her to identify with him. Therefore, blind to any common ground she and her patient may share, the psychiatrist can fall into the trap of easing or forcing her crazy patient into a more familiar category: my patient is ill, he needs to be cared for by me, a doctor; if he doesn't agree, I must remove his civil rights so he will be obliged to accept the patient role. The mad person's unconventional way of life is his taste—habit? preference? deed? speech?—not to my taste and probably not to yours, but to his. Unless he breaks the law or trespasses on the psychiatrist's person, I see no reason for any reaction other than tolerance and a willingness to help. But it's hard to let people be.

Were my imperfect dream for psychiatry to have a happy outcome (an outcome in which psychiatrists think darkly and contemplatively, take on mysteries in the style of women, cast doubt on clarity as German philosophers do, and, like Russian novelists, devote more attention to misery), I'd still be a peddler of doom and gloom. Would ordinary citizens, I wonder, deprived of the easy-to-scapegoat category of people called "the mad," find new categories of people to scapegoat—Muslims, Martians, or Muscovites, perhaps? Our penchant for debasing those unlike ourselves—I wish this weren't true—sometimes looks intractable, and villainous leaders capitalize on this. Wicked self-assigned messiahs propagandize hatred against the outsider, scapegoating and mistreating any tribe or subgroup that, even in a trivial way, is different—skin colour, gender, cultural differences, and for psychiatrists, behavioural differences. The crueller and more honest language is that we—all of us—*have a penchant for* and *latch onto* villainous leaders and villainous culture heroes, icons who legitimize our frightening tendency to be mean and to be prejudiced. We humans are nasty, ready to hate, blame, and persecute, and yes, to rape, pillage, and murder.

A trivial example is when I can't find something on my desk; despite our thirty years together, it's always my housecleaner Alcina's fault. The serious examples are tribal—our readiness to cheer George W. Bush's attack on Iraq, then a few months later, our disgust with those "stupid Americans" for their country's attack on Iraq. Let's be dead honest—we are all frustrated by damned Americans, damned Muslims, damned French, Christians, Israelis, Africans—and so on forever.

Let me tell a cautionary tale, a reminder that we all know things we don't want to know. Tyrants like Hitler and Stalin spring up from time to time, and they always will. Yet Hitler and Stalin aren't the only ones who worry me. I also worry about me . . . and you. But let me start with the Germans. Why were they silent when it was obvious Hitler was a diabolical killer? They'd seen what was going on. They knew their friends were taken away. Soldiers on leave would have told their wives what was going on in the extermination camps. In 1941, my Uncle Ernst, who lived in Vienna, was drinking with his friends at his *Stammtisch* (his regular table at his regular club, with close friends) one night and boisterously announced that "*Der Hitler ist ein Arschloch!*" (Hitler is an asshole)—to great hilarity. Within days, he was in Dachau (at the same time another uncle was in the Canadian navy and my father in an internment camp in Canada). But while most Germans knew that Ernst was right, that Hitler was an asshole, few did anything about it.

Uncle Ernst's son, my cousin Alwin, is gay, physically small, and very effeminate. Because he is Viennese, he thinks like a Latin, emotional and effusive, and when he visits, he wants to hug me. My family is from northern Germany, and my tastes, "sensible" like the English, Swedes, and Germans, are more reserved, so when Alwin wants to hug I'm hyper-alert. He, of course, aims his lips directly at my lips, so I have to move fast to escape—usually by a whisker. When drafted by the *Wehrmacht* during World War II, Alwin twice got himself kicked out for bedwetting and some other contrived limitation, but when drafted a third time, he finally deserted. Despite the Nazi era, my guess is that in Germany, even today, a German soldier who deserted is not a hero. Because he wasn't a Hollywood hero, Alwin's story is problematic; I expect that those who know of what happened think of him as a coward and a sissy. But he did stand for a principle, in his case, outrage that the government would inflict on him the indignity of being a soldier. Most in Germany weren't indignant, even if they had grounds worthier than Alwin's; they were silent. A question looms and weighs on me: Had I lived in Germany during World War II, would I have held my tongue? Of all the horrors, the most worrisome is the great silence. A woman interviewed on the streets of New York was asked whether she was troubled that George W. Bush had authorized torturing prisoners. Her reply: "He's the commander-in-chief." The psychiatric equivalent of this would be, "Well, that's the modern psychiatric treatment." Seeing that people think this way is what makes me worry about me... and you.

The stories of *Tess of the d'Urbervilles* and of Marilyn Monroe are tragic but also thrilling, but we aren't supposed to admit to the thrilling part, that we humans are interested in macabre, disturbing things like suicide, mass killings, sexual exploitation, and hysterical naïveté (although the media don't hesitate to use this interest for their purposes). Most of us laugh at *America's Funniest Home Videos*, even though the humour is always a sadistic response to someone's pratfall, to people who've failed, been humiliated, or even injured. Psychiatrists often see and have to work with this awful thinking—doctors who God, fate, or destiny assigned to do this job. For now, the rapture/dismay of insight—especially insight into our own intestines and our own nastiness—are it, *it* being the current way of practising, however tentative a fashion it may turn out to be. It may be different tomorrow.

22
A Satire

The satirist is harsher [than the ironist], employing ridicule, contempt, indignation, anger; his attack is "grounded in ethical standards"; he is a moralist.
D.J. ENRIGHT

I'VE HAD A good visit in Mexico and, like Anneliese Muther in my office and Hans Castorp in *The Magic Mountain*, I've watched and pondered, amazed at human shenanigans, yet not amazed at all. At the end of my trip, I'm back where I started—bewildered, amused, bemused, worried, still plagued by utopianism, unable to keep in mind that getting things straight once and for all is only a daydream. Watching has been fun, but writing this book has been a brawl. Like the wars between Settembrini and Naphta on Thomas Mann's magic mountain, it's been a fight to the finish with my psychiatric forebears and many modern colleagues. And now I'm in the departure lounge waiting for my Air Canada flight at the Aeropuerto Benito Juarez in Mexico City, heading for home—and still watching. It would be fitting if I were to arrive at a conclusion while still in Mexico. And here it is: psychiatrists are fixated on a hopeful but dangerous miscalculation.

The couple beside me are hugging, holding a camera, both laughing at a photo she's just taken. And because she is leaving him behind, both are brushing away tears. They are doing what we all do: mirror-play with a photograph, adding one more flickering duplicate to a billion duplicates already on record, words and images, good and bad, timeless and indelible. From Nietzsche, I learned that "madness is rare in individuals, but in groups, parties, nations, and ages, it is the rule," so, since the couple are a group of two, I imagine they are having a small madness together. When I'm in psychiatric mode, I'm inclined to say there are no individuals, that all of us are inextricably bound to others, which means I can pretend Nietzsche was wrong: every one of us communes with the loved and the hated, with the lost, gone, and absent, a community fashioned out of dreams, a metropolis that includes the many never met. And if Nietzsche is wrong, if we never escape from family, tribe, group, party, nation, and era, then we are all destined to be mad, gloriously or horribly mad—or both.

Across from me in the departure lounge is a Hasidic Jew, davening gently and studying his little book. He is dressed in traditional garb except that he isn't wearing a coat and—this strikes me as odd—over his tasselled vest he wears a heavy white Indian sweater decorated with reindeer, a difference from the attire I've previously seen among the Hasidim. The scene conjures up another departure lounge, this one in Vienna a few years ago. At the gate beside mine was a group of nine or ten men who reminded me of Nietzsche's aphorism about madness in groups being the rule. All were remarkably crazy, each afflicted with an identical form of schizophrenia, yet they were scheduled to board a flight to Kiev. Their bizarre behaviour was a dead giveaway. I was quite taken aback. They were identically dressed in black suits, old-fashioned black overcoats, and black broad-brimmed fedoras. All had beards and dangling curls in front of their ears, like the ringlets worn by schoolgirls when I was a boy. The mirror-play was extreme; each looked just like his fellows.

I've encountered many schizophrenics, but never before in a group, all with the same symptom picture, so I watched carefully. The other passengers had already boarded and the staff tried to get these men to board the plane, but despite the last call announcement, they wouldn't cooperate. They were in good spirits, laughing and horsing around, and since they were delaying the flight, their carefree (careless?) attitude was surprising: *inappropriate affect* is the psychiatric term. They seemed to be under a group delusion as they walked toward the windows that overlooked the tarmac. Such self-centredness is common in schizophrenia, the medical term being *narcissism*.

The men removed their coats and fedoras, and each opened a kit or case from which they removed blocks (of wood?) encased in leather before attaching these to their foreheads with a strap. With another set of straps, each wrapped his left forearm and upper arm. They were skilful at getting these things in place, indicating they'd practised this bizarre behaviour many times. Finally, they draped decorated shawls across their shoulders before pulling one edge over the tops of their heads, creating a sort of hood. Rhythmically swaying and bobbing their heads, they approached the window, peered into small books, and mumbled something, almost a chant. Then, as quickly as they'd begun, they dismantled everything and packed up.

Next, one of them took another by the hand and insisted they dance sideways along the aisle between the departure lounge seats. His partner laughed and went along with this for thirty seconds or so. I suspect this was some kind of feminine thing, an obliviousness to the fact that men do not usually dance together. I noticed another feminine gesture—tugging at and playing with the curls that hung down the sides of their faces. It seemed clear that there was some kind of delusional system behind all this. I'd certainly have liked to interview them. It wasn't their bizarre behaviour or their delusions that interested me—I'm used to schizophrenic behaviour in hospitals—but the fact that they were schizophrenic in unison, an unusual and rare form of the disease. There are cases of *folie à deux*, of course, but I've never heard of a joint psychosis shared by more than two people (even that is rare). A group as large as this is unheard of. These men ought to be studied. I'd suggest routine things be done—EEGs, X-rays, brain imaging, probably in a hospital—both for their own protection and to be sure we could get the investigations done.

YES, MADNESS—HUMAN LIFE, in other words—is everywhere: tallit, tefillin, phylacteries, circumcision, crucifixes, bishops' mitres, nuns' habits, turbans, head scarves, purple Mohawk haircuts, rap gangster clothes, tattoos, body piercings, high heels, tai chi, snake oil, my Rolex watch, dietary fads, abstract art, and Hasidic Jews boarding an airplane, not to speak of people lying on psychiatrists' couches. But I strongly recommend that you do none of these things on your own. If it's not the custom of a group, you'll be pronounced a madman. Why, I ask, is uniqueness intolerable, but the oddness of a group okay?

To follow public opinion is to be drunk—with obedience. It's no sin to be drunk with hope, fear, or Canadian Club whiskey, but respect for the insane demands that we become drunk many times over, especially with points of view that force us to let go of blind orthodoxy. Such intoxications, well indulged, make us, if not serene, at least tolerant. They make it possible to treat crazy people respectfully—succour them, order them around, listen to their stories, yell when they are stupid, share a few laughs, and give them a pill now and then.

> Somewhere in Pennsylvania, Anne Merak works as an assistant to the sun. She's been in that line of work for as long as she can recall. At the end of every night, Anne raises her arms and pushes the sun up into the sky. Lowering her arms at the day's end she puts the sun down to bed on the horizon. She was very small when she started this job, and she's never missed a shift. Half a century ago, she was declared insane. Since then Anne has gone through several institutions, been treated by numerous psychiatrists, and swallowed innumerable pills. They never managed to cure her.
>
> Thank heavens.[1]

My allotted time is done, so it's time to take leave of psychiatry's howling confusions—of my amazing Vanity Fair. Now that my visit is over, after tedious arguments and insidious intent, in the room the women still come and go, talking of Michelangelo—which leads to a strong conclusion:

All human actions—including the ministrations of shamans and priests—are deeply ritualized biography and superstition.

---

1 Eduardo Galeano, "Sun," in *Voices of Time: A Life in Stories* (New York: Picador, 2007).

Acknowledgements

I WANT TO thank my editor, Arlene Prunkl, for her critical comments and corrections. Without her help, this would have been a lesser book.

I'm grateful to the Ontario Council for the Arts for their financial support.

Made in the USA
Monee, IL
05 November 2026

68006392R00163